INTRODUCTION TO PATHOLOGY
FOR RADIOGRAPHERS

INTRODUCTION TO
PATHOLOGY
FOR
RADIOGRAPHERS

NEIL PRIME DCR(R)

Superintendent I Radiographer
Brook General Hospital
London

Harper & Row, Publishers
London

Cambridge
Mexico City
New York
Philadelphia

San Francisco
São Paulo
Singapore
Sydney

I would like to dedicate
this book to Helen

First published 1987

Harper & Row Ltd
28 Tavistock Street
London WC2E 7PN

British Library Cataloguing in Publication Data
Prime, Neil
  Introduction to pathology for
  radiographers.
  1. Pathology
  I. Title
  616.07′024616   RB111

ISBN 0–06–318362–5

Typeset by Bookworm Typesetting, Manchester
Printed and bound by Butler & Tanner Ltd, Frome and London

CONTENTS

Preface   vi

Acknowledgements   vii

1 General pathology   1
2 Diseases of the lung and respiratory system   11
3 Diseases of the cardiovascular system   44
4 Diseases of the blood   77
5 Diseases of the digestive system   97
6 Hepatobiliary system diseases including the pancreas   128
7 Lymphatic system diseases including the breast   144
8 Diseases of the nervous system including the eye and ear   153
9 Skin, connective tissue and muscle diseases   193
10 Diseases of the urino-genital system   203
11 Bone and joint disease   241
12 Fractures   266
13 Diseases of the endocrine system   295

Glossary   314

Bibliography   319

Index   321

PREFACE

This book has been written as an introduction to pathology for both students and qualified radiographers. It is not a comprehensive study of this vast subject, but I hope it will act as a starting point for those interested in finding out more about this essential subject.

The radiographs included are used to illustrate the most common pathology encountered by diagnostic radiographers in their day-to-day work. More complicated radiographs can be found in more complex texts. The illustrations have been prepared to show both normal and abnormal pathology.

ACKNOWLEDGEMENTS

I have many people to thank for helping me compile this book. They include: Barry Thomas, Keith Stean, Andy Martin, Dr A. Sandhu, Dr R. B. Sakya, Dr J. M. C. Walfula, Dr M. Michelle, Dai Davies and the staff of Brook General Hospital X-ray Department.

The illustrations have been drawn by K. Davidson DCR(R).

1
GENERAL PATHOLOGY

This opening chapter is written as an introduction to some aspects of general pathology and gives an outline of the following areas:

(1) Tumours.
(2) Infection and disease.
(3) Bacteria.
(4) Viruses.

DEFINITIONS

Pathology

Pathology is the study of disease and the process of disease.

Types of disease

(1) Inherited. This is a disease that is passed from one or both parents to the child, e.g. haemophilia.
(2) Congenital. This is an abnormality that is present at birth, but which is not genetically determined. The condition is acquired in utero, e.g. congenital dislocation of the hips (CDH).
(3) Acquired. This is a disease that occurs through a response to the presence of a stimulus. This includes infection with bacteria, viruses and tumours.

TUMOURS

A tumour or neoplasm is an abnormal mass of tissue or an abnormal cell population. A tumour is usually characterized by an excessive proliferation of cells that is beyond the physiological demands of the organ or organs involved.

Characteristics of a tumour

Site

Tumours may arise anywhere within the body. It is generally accepted that more superficial tumours have a better prognosis.

Size

The size of tumours varies widely. The size of the tumour has no bearing upon its prognosis. Large does not mean a poor result. With better health care and health education, tumours are being detected and diagnosed at a much earlier stage.

Shape

The tumour usually adopts the basic structure of the area in which it is growing. Superficial skin tumours have a varied appearance and shape. Tumours growing inside structures, e.g. the ventricles of the brain, are limited in their growth by the skull and tend to adopt the shape of the ventricle.

Capsule

Tumours may be surrounded by a well-formed capsule. Other types have no capsule and tend to be more invasive.

Cell pattern

Tumour cells are often similar to the tissues from which they are growing. It is usually found that tumours with cell patterns most different from the tissue of origin are the more aggressive.

Benign or malignant

This is the most important characteristic of a tumour, and classification of the tumour into benign or malignant is made on the following characteristics:

Benign

(1) Growth is usually very slow. The tumour may grow for many years before becoming apparent. Some tumours may cease to grow at a certain point.
(2) Benign tumours are usually encapsulated.
(3) They grow by expansion of the surrounding tissues.
(4) They remain localized to the tissue or organ of origin.
(5) The tumour tissue is usually similar to the tissue of origin.
(6) There is little or no destruction of normal tissue.
(7) Benign tumours are usually not fatal. Benign tumours may prove fatal if they compress certain vital sites, e.g. the bronchus. Some tumours may disrupt endocrine gland function, e.g. pituitary adenomas.

Malignant

(1) Rate of growth is variable and may be very rapid. There is a non-uniform rate of growth of the tumour.
(2) Usually not encapsulated.
(3) Grow by infiltration of surrounding tissues.
(4) The tumour spreads from the initial site (primary growth) to other sites via secondary spread (metastasis). This may be via the blood, lymphatic system, cerebrospinal fluid, etc. Malignant tumours always spread.
(5) Histology usually diverges widely from the tissue of origin, particularly at later stages. Very poorly differentiated malignant tumours are called anaplastic.
(6) Causes destruction of surrounding tissue. This is extensive at later stages.
(7) Fatal if untreated. The tumour may be difficult to treat due to secondary spread.

Classification of tumours

Many systems of tumour classification have been proposed. One tumour classification is based upon a combination of:

(1) Histogenesis or tissue of origin.
(2) Histology or tissue type within the tumour.
(3) Behaviour.

Tumours of epithelial tissue

Benign tumours of epithelial origin are given the suffix *-oma,* whereas malignant tumours of epithelial origin are given the suffix *-carcinoma.*

Table 1.1 Classification of tumours

	Benign	Malignant
(1) *Epithelium*		
	Squamous papilloma	Squamous-cell carcinoma
	Transitional papilloma	Transitional cell carcinoma
Glandular:		
Papillary	Papilloma	Papillary carcinoma
Solid	Adenoma	Adenocarcinoma
Cystic	Cystadenoma	Cystadenocarcinoma
Mixed cystic papillary, papillary and papillary cystadenoma, cystadenocarcinoma		
(2) *Connective and supportive tissues*		
Fibrous tissue	Fibroma	Fibrosarcoma
Cartilage	Chondroma	Chondrosarcoma
Bone	Osteoma	Osteosarcoma
Adipose tissue	Lipoma	Liposarcoma
Blood vessels	Haemangioma	Haemangiosarcoma
(3) *Muscle*		
Smooth	Leiomyoma	Leiomyosarcoma
Striated	Rhabdomyoma	Rhabdomyosarcoma
(4) *Nervous tissue*		
Glial tissue	Glioma	
Nerve sheath	Neurilemoma	Neurogenic sarcoma
Meninges	Meningioma	Meningeal sarcoma
Peripheral nerve cells	Ganglioneuroma	
	Neuroblastoma	
(5) *Reticuloendothelial tissue*		
Lymphoid tissue		Hodgkin's lymphoma, non-Hodgkin's lymphoma
Granulocytes		Myeloid leukaemia
Plasma cells		Myeloma
(6) *Tumours of childhood*		
	Neuroblastoma	
	Retinoblastoma	
	Nephroblastoma	

A benign tumour of a surface epithelium is called a papilloma, whereas one of glandular origin is called an adenoma. Adenomas may also be cystic and are then called cystadenomas. A malignant epithelial tumour of glandular origin is called an adenocarcinoma. Carcinomas of surface epithelial origin are usually further classified by adding the cell origin of the tumour, e.g. squamous-cell carcinoma.

Tumours of connective tissue

Benign tumours of connective tissues are given the suffix *-oma*. Malignant tumours of connective tissue are classified by the suffix *-sarcoma*. The tumours are further categorized by their tissue of origin, e.g. osteoma, osteosarcoma.

Tumours of other tissues, e.g. muscle, are classified as shown in Table 1.1. Greater detail of individual tumours is given in later chapters.

Methods of spread

A number of routes of spread are available for the dissipation of metastasise from the primary growth. Benign tumours remain localized and spread locally.

Direct spread

Direct spread of a tumour relies upon the rate at which the cells within the tumour are multiplying, and the motility of the tumour cells.

Spread of malignant tumours may occur through:

(1) Direct.
(2) Lymph.
(3) Blood.
(4) Transcoelomic.
(5) Implantation.

Routes of direct spread

(1) Tissue spaces. Tumour cells tend to take the path of least resistance and will attempt to move along the lines of anatomical cleavage. Later growth of the tumour becomes less well defined.
(2) Lymphatic vessels. Tumour cells may spread along lymphatic vessels.
(3) Veins. Tumours may also spread into and along veins. This usually occurs after lymphatic spread. Invasion of arteries is less common due to the thickness and pulsation of arterial walls and the velocity of arterial blood.
(4) Epithelial cavities. Direct invasion of cavities, e.g. bladder, sinuses.

Lymph spread

Tumour cells may spread by permeation throughout the lymphatic system. Lymph nodes allow the growth of tumour cells. Secondary tumour growth may occur from lymph nodes following removal of the primary tumour.

Blood spread (haematogenic)

Blood spread usually results from invasion of the venous or lymphatic system. Lymph containing metastases or tumour emboli may be passed into the venous system. Blood-borne tumour emboli are initially carried to the capillary system. From here they most commonly lodge in the brain, lungs and liver. If the transported embolus survives, a secondary tumour forms.

Transcoelomic spread

This may occur through shedding of malignant cells into the peritoneum or pleura.

Malignant spread through the peritoneum may arise from the ovary or bowel. Spread through the peritoneum may be controlled by gravity with the downward movement of metastasise.

Spread into the pericardium is uncommon.

Transcoelomic spread may result in effusion. This is an inflammatory response to the presence of metastasise. This results in vascular and lymphatic obstruction and ascites. Adhesion of structures may also result together with invasion of the viscera.

Implantation

Spread of metatasise may occur through:

(1) Spread via natural pathways, e.g. respiratory tract, urinary tract.
(2) Surgical transplantation. Removal of tumours may result in spillage of tumour cells. This is overcome by microsurgical techniques. Needle biopsy of tumours must be carefully carried out to avoid spread through other tissue layers.

Grading of tumours

Usually malignant tumours are graded, by using Roman numerals, into three or four grades (I-IV). The higher numbers indicate more advanced tumours with a poorer prognosis. Grading is therefore important for prognosis. Three factors are considered in cancer grading:

(1) Degree of tissue differentiation.
(2) Estimated growth rate.
(3) Type of cells present.

INFECTION AND DISEASE

The source of infection

The source of an infection is the site from where the pathogen is growing. Infection in man may be autogenous (self-infection) or exogenous where infection is from another source.

Autogenous source

This involves spread of infection from one part of the body to another. This may occur by:

(1) Direct contact. Thus the bacteria *Escherichia coli* (*E. coli*) may be spread from the bowel via the anus to the urinary tract.
(2) Blood-borne. The infection may also be spread via the bloodstream. Extraction of a chronically infected tooth may result in the spread of infection to other parts of the body (e.g. *Streptococcus viridans.*) If the organism lodges in the heart, this can cause extensive heart valve disease.

Exogenous source

Infection from other sources may be spread in a variety of ways:

(1) Direct route. Direct contact between people may result in the spread of infection.
(2) Indirect route. This involves spread of infection from the area of infection to the patient without direct contact.

Methods of indirect spread include:

(1) Airborne infection. This is transmitted by droplets exhaled from the nose and upper airway, and by dust particles. Some bacteria, e.g. the streptococci, are capable of surviving in dust for extended periods of time. Thus adequate and regular cleaning of the radiography department must be carried out.
(2) Fomites (inanimate objects). Spread of infection from fomites, e.g. from contaminated drinking glasses to the patient, is another common route of infection. Cleaning of work surfaces and equipment is therefore important.
(3) Blood and food-borne infection causes ingestion of infected materials. This may occur through poor hygiene, contamination of water supplies or contamination of food via insects. Ingestion usually causes extensive systemic infections.

(4) Infection from instruments. Infection may be spread from contaminated instruments, e.g. needles. There is an increased risk of infection via this route in hospitals. Spread of hepatitis B due to poor handling of infected syringes must be avoided.

BACTERIAL INFECTIONS

The majority of bacteria are unicellular organisms, although they may be found as clusters, chains or collections of filaments. Figure 1.1 shows types of bacteria.

Most bacteria exist independently of a living host and are called saprophytes. Others rely for their survival by existing on or in a living host. These are called parasites. The parasitic bacteria may be further divided into:

(1) Commensals. These co-exist with the host cells and cause no disruption to their function.
(2) Pathogens. These invade and cause damage to the host. Commensals may invade the host and become pathogens if the cell barrier is broken. This may happen following an injury to the skin, where invasion of the wound by bacteria may take place.
(3) Anaerobic. This type of bacteria cannot survive in the presence of oxygen.
(4) Aerobic. These rely on oxygen for their survival.

Classification of bacteria is made in a variety of ways, for instance on the

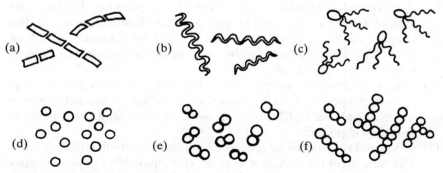

Figure 1.1 Types of bacteria: (a) bacilli; (b) spirochaete; (c) flagellae; (d) staphylococci; (e) pneumococci and (f) streptococci

way in which a bacteria reacts to particular stains. Bacteria cause disruption to the host cells by:

(1) Their ability to break down the local defense mechanisms. This is achieved through the release of enzymes and other chemicals that disrupt cell membranes. In severe cases bacteria may infect the bloodstream and multiply freely, forming a septicaemia.
(2) By the release of toxins. Endotoxins are retained by the cell and are released when the bacteria dies. Exotoxins are released by multiplying bacteria.

Table 1.2 Examples of bacterial infections

Type of bacteria	Disease
Streptococcus viridans	Subacute bacterial endocarditis (SBE)
Streptococcus pyogenes	Infection of wounds
Streptococcus pneumoniae	Lobar pneumonia
Clostridium perfringens	Gas gangrene
Staphylococcus aureus	Osteomyelitis
Haemophilus influenzae	Chronic bronchitis
Escherichia coli	Septicaemia
Salmonella typhi	Typhoid fever
Mycobacterium tuberculosis	Tuberculosis

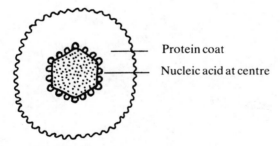

Protein coat

Nucleic acid at centre

Figure 1.2 Diagram of a virus

VIRUSES

Viruses are small infectious agents of variable size (approximately 20–400 nm). They are composed of a central core of nucleic acid surrounded by a protein coat (capsid) (Figure 1.2). This simple structural unit is called the virion.

Viruses are classified by the type of nucleic acid they contain. This may be either ribonucleic acid (RNA) or deoxyribonucleic acid (DNA). RNA-type viruses include the rhinoviruses that cause the common cold; DNA viruses include the herpes viruses that cause herpes simplex.

Other diseases caused by viral infection include: measles, mumps, German measles and acquired immune deficiency syndrome (AIDS) or human immuno deficiency virus (HIV).

2
DISEASES OF THE LUNG
AND RESPIRATORY SYSTEM

THE NOSE

The nose allows air into and protects the respiratory system, both warming and filtering the air before it reaches the lungs. It also keeps the inspired air moist to protect the surfaces where gaseous exchange takes place. The nose is the first line of defence, and is open to a wide range of infections.

Acute rhinitis

This is an inflammation of the nasal mucosa caused by virus or allergy. The condition is characterized by swelling of the mucosa and the release of a watery exudate. Viruses are known to cause rhinitis. These include the rhinoviruses of which there are approximately ninety types.

NASOPHARYNX

The nasopharynx may be radiographed in children to show the extent of the adenoids. This is tissue of lymphatic origin that may become enlarged in response to a generalized infection of the nose and upper respiratory tract.

THE PARANASAL SINUSES

The paranasal sinuses freely communicate with the nasal cavity and allow the passage of infection between them. The sinuses are lined by a thin layer of mucosa. Radiographs of the sinuses demonstrate the mucosa when it is inflammed.

Sinusitis

Sinusitis presents in a similar way to rhinitis with bacterial or viral infiltration causing inflammation of the mucosa. The maxillary antra is the sinus most commonly affected. Sinusitis may also be caused by:

(1) Infection of the maxillary sinuses following the extraction of teeth. The roots of the teeth may pass into the antra causing widespread infections. The sinuses may be radiographed to show retained roots.
(2) Production of large amounts of mucus may cause blockage of the sinuses, which may lead to chronic infection. This can be demonstrated as an opaque sinus or as a fluid level within the sinus depending upon the extent of the blockage and the stage of the infection. If left untreated, infected material may pass into the thin walls of the sinuses causing osteomyelitis of the skull. Benign cystic lesions of the sinuses may also develop and occlude proper drainage.

Polyps

Polyps are outgrowths of the mucosa of the sinuses or the nose. They are not true tumours and are thought to occur due to long-standing allergic rhinitis caused by, e.g. house dust, mites, animal products. Polyps may obstruct the drainage passages of the nose and sinuses causing sinusitis.

Tumours of the upper respiratory tract

Haemangioma (angiofibroma)

This is a vascular tumour that may appear in the nose. It may rupture and bleed extensively and can be treated by embolisation of the lesion under radiographic control.

Papilloma

This benign tumour may be found in the nose or the sinuses. The tumour may cause blockage of the nose and sinuses.

Carcinomas

The commonest carcinomas of the upper respiratory tract are of the squamous cell type. Spread is usually by direct infiltration of adjacent structures. Surgical removal of the tumour produces a very low survival rate due to the difficulties encountered in removing the entire tumour.

THE LARYNX

The larynx protects the respiratory tract against inhalation of food, vomit, etc. The cough reflex helps to expel harmful substances.

The larynx is commonly involved when the nose and sinuses become infected. Laryngitis or laryngeal swelling may follow the common cold or influenza. This swelling may cause compression of the airway.

Diphtheria (*Corynebacterium diphtheriae*) was once a common infection of the larynx and pharynx. This disease has now been controlled following widespread inoculation.

Carcinoma of the larynx

Carcinoma of the larynx accounts for 1 per cent of all deaths due to malignancy per year in England and Wales. The carcinoma develops in two ways:

(1) Intrinsic carcinomas. This is the commonest form arising directly from the vocal chords.
(2) Extrinsic carcinomas are less common and arise from structures adjacent to the larynx, e.g. the epiglottis.

The tumour spreads initially by local invasion upward and sideways. The intrinsic type remains localized for long periods, but the extrinsic type is more vigorous. At a later stage the tumour will spread eventually through the lymphatic system and become blood-borne.

THE CHEST

Anatomy of the lungs

The lungs are divided into lobes (Figure 2.1). There are three lobes on the right and two on the left. The lungs are covered by the pleura, which follows the lines of the lobes. The lobes are subdivided by septa into bronchopulmonary segments. The bronchi subdivide to form bronchioles, which further subdivide to form alveoli. Each lobe is supplied by a branch of the bronchus.

Signs and symptoms of chest disease

(1) Clubbing. Clubbing (Figure 2.2) of the fingers is associated with a variety of chest complaints, e.g. congenital heart abnormalities, bronchial carcinoma and bronchiectasis. On inspection of the hands,

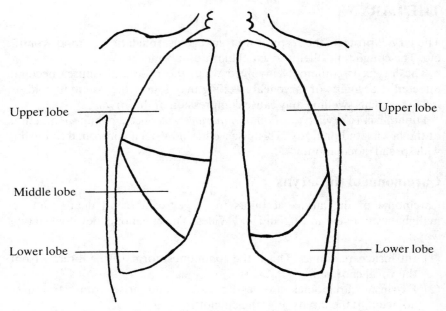

Figure 2.1 Basic anatomy: the lobes of the lungs, anterior aspect

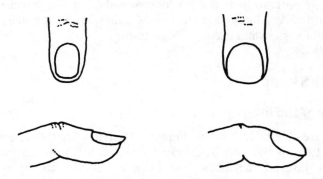

Figure 2.2 Finger clubbing: normal (left) and clubbed finger with distorted nail (right)

the nails appear more rounded and the nail bed is raised.
(2) Cyanosis. Peripheral cyanosis affects the limbs and may be due to localized circulatory problems. Central cyanosis implies that there is improper oxygenation due to disease of the blood in the heart and lungs.

(3) Breathing. The respiratory rate and the manner of breathing may also indicate the presence of disease. Breathlessness (dyspnoea) is associated with pneumothorax, effusions, pneumonia.
(4) Sputum. Sputum production is always indicative of disease. Serous sputum is non-infected. Purulent sputum describes infected sputum and indicates the presence of bacteria. The amount and type of purulent sputum indicates the stage and extent of the disease.
(5) Haemoptysis. The coughing up of blood requires thorough investigation. The colour and amount of the blood indicates the region from which blood has come. Loss of large amounts of blood through coughing indicates pulmonary infarction whereas small flecks of blood within the sputum may indicate bronchial carcinoma.

Pneumonia

Pneumonia (Figure 2.3) is a general term used to describe an inflammation of the lung tissue. The infection causes an inflammatory reaction with the subsequent release of exudate into the alveoli, which produces consolidation within the lungs.

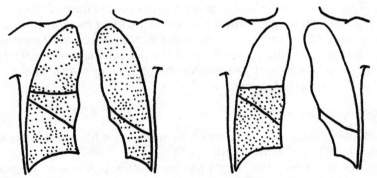

Figure 2.3 Types of pneumonia: bronchopneumonia (left) and lobar pneumonia (right)

Causes

Pneumonia is caused by a range of bacteria and frequently occurs as a complication of another disease. Age and previous health of the patient may determine the type of severity of pneumonia. The commonest causes of pneumonia are:

(1) Virus.
(2) *Streptococcus pneumoniae.*
(3) *Staphylococcus pyogenes.*
(4) *Escherichia coli.*
(5) *Legionella pneumophilia* (Legionnaire's disease).

Elderly patients, neonates and patients on assisted ventilation, unless properly managed, are prone to pnuemonia.

Types

Pneumonia can be subdivided into two main types:

(1) Lobar pneumonia. This describes a pneumonia restricted to one or more discrete lobes.
(2) Bronchopneumonia. This type of pneumonia is characterized by a patchy involvement of the whole lung tissue.

Lobar

Lobar pneumonia is commonest in young healthy adults and is caused by pneumococci- or streptococci-type bacteria. Legionella virus may also cause lobar pneumonia.

The pneumonia develops quickly, often with no apparent underlying cause. As the disease develops the inhaled bacteria cause the release of exudate. Sputum may be stained with blood. The chest radiograph shows the infection to be restricted to a single discrete lobe, or, rarely, to multiple lobes. The lobe appears dense and opaque due to consolidation of the lobe. Pus does not usually form in pneumococcal lobar pneumonia.

The pneumonia is treated by antibiotics with good results. The exudate is absorbed by the walls of the alveoli as the pneumonia resolves. Delayed or incomplete healing may produce fibrosis of the lung tissue. This may be noted on follow-up radiographs.

Bronchopneumonia

Bronchopneumonia is more common than the lobar form and is the most common form found in the elderly.

Diseases that lower the body's immunity often give rise to bronchopneumonia. Staphylococci, pneumococci and viruses can all cause bronchopneumonia. The disease is characterized by being dispersed throughout the lung and is commonly bilateral, lying in the lower portion of the lungs. The alveoli become filled with exudate, which prevents drainage. Pus builds up in the infected areas. The destruction of lung tissue differentiates bronchopulmonary pneumonia from the lobar type.

Commonly the patient has a productive cough with a raised temperature and purulent sputum.

Bronchopneumonia is a more chronic condition than lobar pneumonia. The disease may also be complicated by extensive destruction of the lung tissue and the formation of abscesses. Bronchopneumonia is also a frequent cause of death and is commonly associated with the terminal stage of disease.

Other types

Legionella (Legionnaire's disease)

This is due to *Legionella pneumophila* and gives rise to severe illness and may result in death. The illness occurs in epidemics and produces lobar-type pneumonias. The pneumonia is severe and causes extensive damage to the lungs.

Aspiration pneumonia

This occurs following aspiration of food, gastric contents containing hydrochloric acid or other infected material into the lungs. Should the aspirated material occlude a lobar bronchus, this will cause lobar consolidation. If it is distributed in scattered bronchial segments this may cause bronchopneumonia.

Aspiration of the gastric contents causes widespread damage of the alveoli. Undigested particles of food will act as foci for the disease.

The condition may develop through severe gastro-oesophageal reflux, oesophageal diverticula or overspill of the gastric contents following drug overdose, alcohol abuse, anaesthesia or coma.

Other causes

Pneumonia also occurs through:

(1) Fungi, e.g. aspergillus.
(2) Chemicals, e.g. chlorine gas.

Lung abscess

Lung abscesses (Plate 1) are localized suppurative lesions that cause obstruction of the lung parenchyma. The abscess cavity is pus-filled and surrounded by fibrous tissue. Abscess cavity formation is called cavitation. These abscesses can be caused by:

(1) Aspiration of infected material into the lungs. This may occur when the upper respiratory tract and sinuses are infected. The right lung is more prone to infection because the right bronchial division is much shorter than the left.

Abscess due to aspiration of vomit in the supine position may occur in the apical segments of the lower lobes or the posterior segments of the upper lobes. Areas of lung tissue are destroyed which leads to

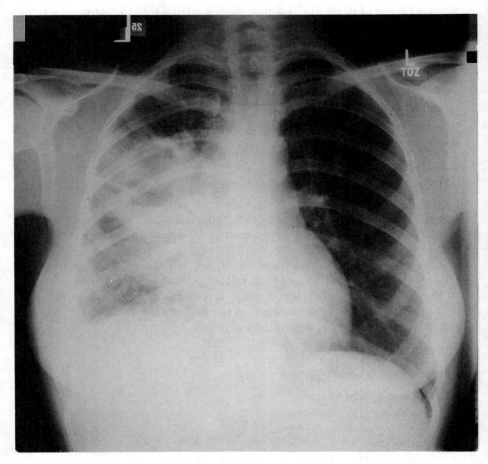

Plate 1   Abscess in the right lung. Note fluid level within the abscess cavity

pneumonia and abscess formation.

(2) Post pneumonia. Abscess cavities may form following bronchopneumonia or lobar pneumonia. The centre of the pneumonia begins to form an abscess, particularly when the pneumonia is caused by staphylococcus or kleibsella bacteria.

(3) Obstruction of the bronchus. Abscess formation may follow obstruction to the bronchus, particularly in cases of carcinoma of the bronchus.

(4) Blood-borne infections. In this case the abscess is usually associated with a recent or ongoing serious illness.

If the abscess cavity communicates with the bronchus, then air will leak into the cavity and the patient will cough up purulent sputum. An erect chest radiograph may show a fluid level within the abscess cavity.

The abscess is treated with antibiotics and may need draining.

Tuberculosis

Tuberculosis (Figure 2.4) in Great Britain is now uncommon. Mortality from the disease in this country is rare, but is much more common in third world countries. The decline of tuberculosis in this country is due to improved techniques in detecting the disease.

Tuberculosis is an infective disease caused by the *Mycobacterium tuberculosis*. Two main types of this bacillus are responsible for causing tuberculosis in man:

(1) The human type – endemic in man.
(2) The bovine type – endemic in cattle.

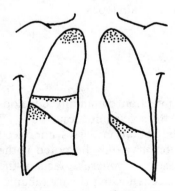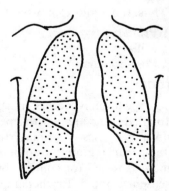

Figure 2.4 Appearances of tuberculosis: confined to apical portions of lobes (left) and miliary tuberculosis (right)

In areas where pasteurization of milk is carried out very little of the bovine type is transmitted.

The characteristic lesion of tuberculosis is the tubercle. This consists of a microscopic collection of epitheloid cells and mycobacterium surrounded by lymphocytes and fibroblasts and is called the Ghon focus.

The initial primary tuberculous infection usually occurs in the lung, but may develop in the alimentary tract. The primary infection or complex is always accompained by regional lymph node involvement. If the primary focus develops in the lung, then the hilar lymph nodes are frequently involved. In the majority of patients the primary infection and associated lymph nodes heal and may calcify. However, in some cases there is delayed healing and spread into the bloodstream occurs. Haemategenous spread of the bacillus may occur to the bones and joints, or to the nervous system, causing tuberculous meningitis.

An unhealed primary pulmonary lesion, particularly when it occurs in adult life, may lead to progressive pulmonary tuberculosis. In advanced cases a tuberculous lesion may rupture through a lymph node into a vein to produce widespread dissemination of the disease. This is called acute miliary tuberculosis and most commonly occurs in children and adolescents.

Progressive pulmonary tuberculosis may occur directly following infection with the bacillus, or much later, following the apparent healing of the disease. This is known as post-primary tuberculosis.

Tuberculosis usually presents with pyrexia, general malaise, loss of appetite, cough with sputum production and, in some cases, haemoptysis. Enlargement of lymph nodes at the time of presentation may also be noted.

Thus, tuberculosis may be classified into three main types:

(1) Primary.
(2) Miliary.
(3) Post-primary.

Primary

This type usually occurs in children. The infection commonly develops through direct contact with a person carrying the active infection.

In many cases of primary tuberculosis the condition passes unnoticed without causing any symptoms. The infection may only be noted if the patient is tested for contact, but in other cases the general effects of the disease are noted. Erythema nodosum is associated with primary tuberculosis and occurs in a number of cases. If the primary focus does not heal the condition may progress to other forms of the disease.

Primary tuberculosis may be diagnosed from culture of bacteria from the patient's sputum, although sputum is often not produced in the primary form. The chest radiograph may show lymph node enlargement. In children, the lymph node enlargement may be pronounced. In adolescents, it may not be so clearly seen. The condition may be complicated by lobe collapse, pneumonia and pleural effusions. Tuberculin testing is used to confirm a suspicion of tuberculosis.

Primary tuberculosis responds well to early treatment with antibiotics.

Miliary

Miliary tuberculosis was once commonly associated with children and young adults. This type of tuberculosis is now becoming more widespread.

The disease may present suddenly, or develop after a few weeks of poor health. The child usually has pyrexia with loss of weight and anaemia. Chest radiographs show characteristic fine mottling of the lung fields. This takes a few weeks to develop and diagnosis is usually confirmed through culture of sputum or tuberculin testing.

The disease responds to antibiotic therapy and is not usually a fatal condition. Complications of the condition include meningitis.

Post-primary

This most commonly occurs in adults. The lesions associated with post-primary tuberculosis commonly develop in the upper lobes or apex of the lower lobes. The lesion usually develops in one lung and spreads to the other via the bronchus.

The disease usually develops slowly with a cough and production of sputum. The chest radiograph may show opacities in the apex of the upper lobes. Calcification may also show through healing of other primary lesions. Cavitation and fibrous tissue formation may also be noted. Cavitation usually indicates active disease. A series of radiographs may be required to show progression of the disease.

If post-primary tuberculosis is suspected sputum culture is usually carried out to confirm diagnosis.

The condition may be complicated by pleurisy or secondary infections of a healed cavity with a fungus such as *Aspergillus fumigatus*. This may be clearly seen on radiographs and is called a mycetoma.

The condition is treated with antibiotic therapy.

Detection

Three to four weeks after initial infection with tuberculosis, the body becomes very sensitive to the protein portion of the tubercle bacillus. This

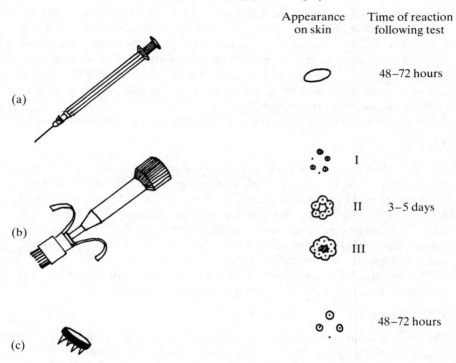

Figure 2.5 Tuberculin testing: (a) Mantoux; (b) Heaf; and (c) Tine

hypersensitivity can be demonstrated with intradermal injections of a purified protein derivative (PPD) of tubercle bacillus, tuberculin testing. The PPD is given in a variety of tests (Figure 2.5):

(1) Mantoux test. In this test a 1:10,000 solution of PPD is injected intradermally. The test is read 48–72 hours later. A positive test with indicated present or past exposure to mycobacterium tuberculosis is indicated by a raised red area of skin at least 10 mm in diameter.
(2) Heaf test. This is the more common type of testing. The Heaf test uses an automatic 'punch gun' that delivers multiple punctures of PPD into the skin. Raised areas of reddened skin around the puncture sites indicates a reaction to the bacillus. The reaction is graded and the most extreme (Grade III) is classed as a positive reaction. The reaction is read after 3–5 days.
(3) Tine test. This uses a disposable tine and is a manual method of conducting the Heaf test. The tine is pressed into the skin. The test is

read after 48–72 hours; 2–4 raised areas around the needle marks of 2–4 mm in diameter are taken as a positive result.

Further tests on sputum are carried out to culture any organisms present.

Treatment

Patients with tuberculosis are isolated from other patients to prevent the spread of infection. This is important to consider when radiographing infected patients.

Known causes of tuberculosis are treated with antibiotics, e.g. streptomycin.

Prophylactic treatment is carried out on children. A BCG (Bacille Calmette-Guérin) injection is given to those children who have given a negative reaction to the Heaf/Mantoux test (tuberculin negative). The BCG injection is given when the child is fourteen years old. A localized skin reaction develops after approximately four weeks. Tuberculin tests after this period give a positive reaction.

Chronic bronchitis and emphysema

Chronic bronchitis and emphysema are often grouped together under the general heading chronic obstructive airways disease (COAD) or chronic obstructive pulmonary disease (COPD). COAD covers a range of conditions extending from pure chronic bronchitis to pure emphysema. Chronic bronchitis and emphysema are usually described separately. Both conditions produce generalized obstruction to the airways and causes widespread pulmonary damage.

Chronic bronchitis

Chronic bronchitis is defined as being a chronic cough with the production of sputum that lasts for three consecutive months in any year for two successive years. Chronic bronchitis frequently occurs with emphysema. Because of this close link, the mixture of emphysema and bronchitis is often referred to as COAD or COPD. This is not a very accurate term because it assumes that emphysema and chronic bronchitis always occur together.

Chronic bronchitis describes a condition which many people develop in response to the long-term action of various types of irritant on the bronchial mucosa. These include:

(1) Cigarette smoking. This is the single most important cause of chronic bronchitis.

(2) Environmental. Air pollution and work-related irritants, e.g. coal dust.
(3) Chronic infections. Long-lasting chronic chest infections may precede bronchitis.

Chronic bronchitis is commoner in middle to late life. It develops slowly and is more common in men than women. The condition is usually worse in the winter months. Irritation of the bronchial mucosa stimulates the mucus-secreting glands in the bronchi and bronchioles to over-secrete. The large amount of mucus produced coats the bronchial walls causing reduction in the area of the air passages, clogging of the bronchioles and obstruction to the movement of air through the airways. Expired air becomes trapped in the alveoli causing them to distend and rupture. The condition is usually complicated by infections that develop due to the poor condition of the cells lining the bronchi. The infection spreads and causes further damage to the lung. Any undamaged alveoli compensate for the damaged lung by enlarging and over-distending. This is called emphysema (see next section).

Patients with chronic bronchitis initially develop a cough, usually in winter, that becomes progressively worse from year to year. Dyspnoea, wheezing and tightness of the chest accompany the cough, and patients produce sputum. This may be clear and copious, or denser and more difficult to clear from the chest by coughing.

This chest condition is treated by:

(1) Removing the bronchial irritant. This usually means encouraging the patient to stop smoking.
(2) Treating underlying chest infections. Sputum from the patient is collected to isolate any bacteria. *Streptococci pneumoniae* is commonly found. The chest infection is treated with antibiotics.

Chronic bronchitis is a progressive disease and requires long-term management. The disease may be complicated by ventilatory and cardiac failure. Patients may survive for up to thirty years of steadily worsening health.

Emphysema

'Emphysema' means an abnormal distension of the tissues with air. This can occur anywhere in the body. For example, penetrating injuries to the chest may cause a pneumothorax and release of air into the subcutaneous tissue around the lung (subcutaneous emphysema). This free air usually tracks upwards into the neck and can be felt below the skin surface.

Surgery may also produce 'surgical emphysema'. This may be seen on the post-operative chest radiographs of patients who have had thoracic surgery as free air in the subcutaneous tissue of the neck and chest. This is absorbed into the tissues with no complications.

Pulmonary emphysema is used to describe emphysematous changes that take place in the lung tissue due to disease.

There are two main types of pulmonary emphysema (Figure 2.6):

(1) Centrilobular. This type of emphysema is associated with chronic bronchitis. There is widespread destruction of the bronchioles due to infections associated with chronic bronchitis. This causes a compensatory over-dilation of undiseased alveoli, such that the walls of the alveoli cannot expand and contract properly. This leads to impaired lung function.

(2) Panacinar emphysema. With this type there is a generalized destruction of the alveolar walls. This type is associated with emphysema as a pure condition. Pulmonary emphysema commonly occurs as a result of chronic bronchitis (COAD) and it is unusual to see emphysema occuring as a distinct condition.

The clinical history of the patient may indicate the type of emphysema present. Pure emphysema is associated with poor ventilatory function early in the disease. The centrilobular type usually occurs in relation to

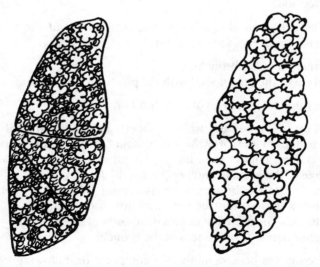

Figure 2.6 Types of emphysema: centrilobular (left) and panacinar (right)

bronchitis with impairment to ventilatory function occurring later in the disease.

Patients with pulmonary emphysema usually complain of dyspnoea on exertion. After walking they breathe heavily to try to compensate for the areas of lung destroyed in emphysema. As the disease progresses the exertional dyspnoea increases and restricts the patient in their movements.

Emphysema is not clearly seen on radiographs of the chest. Changes that may be noted due to emphysema include:

(1) Loss of lung markings.
(2) Low flat diaphragm.
(3) Bullae formation. The lack of normal blood vessels within the lung tissue may become so acute that large air-filled spaces or bullae develop in the lung. These are thin walled structures formed by rupture of the alveolar tissue. They may compress surrounding tissues or rupture causing a pneumothorax.

Respiratory function tests are carried out to help confirm the diagnosis of emphysema.

If the emphysema is associated with chronic bronchitis antibiotic therapy may be given to control underlying chest infections. Physiotherapy may also be necessary to encourage removal of sputum from the chest. Aminophylline, a bronchodilator, may be given in some acute cases.

Bronchiectasis

This is defined as an abnormal permanent dilation of the bronchi. The condition is composed of two elements:

(1) Obstruction of the bronchi.
(2) Infection of the lung tissue, with the production of sputum.

There are three likely causes of the condition:

(1) Build-up of pus due to an underlying infection will cause an obstruction to the bronchi and dilation of the bronchi beyond the obstruction. Unless the site of the infection is cleared widespread damage to the bronchi and permanent dilation will result.
(2) Distension of the bronchi may also result from the formation of pus beyond a lesion obstructing a major bronchus, e.g. a bronchial carcinoma. The infection causes distension of the bronchi.
(3) Congenital mal-development of the bronchi.

The disease was once commonly a complication following measles and whooping cough. The condition is now uncommon due to the widespread use of antibiotics to control infection. Acute pulmony infections in childhood may produce bronchiectasis in adolescence or adulthood.

Bronchiectasis may occur in any part of the lung, although it tends to develop more readily in the middle and lower lobe where drainage of the lung tissue under gravity is not as efficient as in the upper lobe. The patient usually has a chronic cough with the production of purulent sputum. In advanced cases large amounts of sputum are produced. Haemoptysis may also develop due to rupture of vessels within the walls of the alveoli. The sputum may be blood-stained, or there may be large-scale production of blood.

Dilation of the bronchi will not be seen on plain radiographs of the chest.

Bronchography

This is the definitive method of demonstrating bronchiectasis and is one of the very few uses of bronchography. Bronchography is unpleasant and is only used where the diagnosis is not obvious. The areas of the lung most commonly demonstrated as affected are the basal segments of the middle lobe, lower lobe and lingula. The affected areas may appear cylindical, saccular or fusiform.

Sputum

Culture of sputum is always carried out to detect the presence of bacteria.

Due to the over-production of sputum, bronchiectasis may also be associated with chronic bronchitis and pulmonary tuberculosis due to the retention of infection.

Treatment

Bronchiectasis is treated with antibiotics and physiotherapy. Postural drainage may be carried out to promote the production of sputum and thus prevent extensive damage to the lung tissue. Prophylactic treatment may be given to children who have had whooping cough or measles. Surgery may be carried out to remove affected areas of lung.

Cystic fibrosis (mucoviscidosis)

This is an hereditary disease of the exocrine glands. Cystic fibrosis occurs in 1 out of every 2,000 live births. The disease is commoner in Caucasians. The cause of the disease is not fully understood but produces the following effects:

(1) Hypertrophy of mucus-secreting glands.
(2) The lungs are affected in 80–90 per cent of all cases. Widespread

bronchiectasis is noted with chronic chest infections due to the increased production of large amounts of mucus. The mucus is greatly thickened and produced in such large amounts that it is very difficult to remove it from the chest. The sputum is purulent and usually infected with *Staph. aureus*. This infection produces further damage to the lung tissue. As the disease progresses, emphysema develops.

(3) The majority of patients exhibit changes to the pancreas. The gland shrinks and becomes widely replaced by fibrous tissue. The pancreatic ducts become dilated and cystic and fill with mucus secretions. This usually leads to problems of malabsorption. Due to this, patients may appear severely emaciated. The islet cells are usually unaffected.

(4) Chronic obstruction of the liver may be noted. This is due to the increase in viscosity of the bile. Cirrhosis may also develop.

(5) The sweat glands secrete large amounts of sweat containing abnormally high concentrations of sodium and chloride ions. This is due to the sweat glands' inability to reabsorb these elements. Patients with cystic fibrosis are characterized by having excessive sweating.

(6) Males with cystic fibrosis are often sterile due to malformations affecting the vas deferens.

Detection

Approximately half of the cases of cystic fibrosis present themselves in early childhood. The child fails to thrive and exhibits respiratory disorders.

About 10 per cent of cases present at birth with intestinal obstruction that becomes apparent shortly after birth. This obstruction is due to a 'Meconium ileus' and the presence of large amounts of mucus. This is surgically treated in neonates. Another form, 'Meconium ileus equivalent' may occur later in life. This also causes intestinal obstruction but is treated conservatively due to a higher risk of operative mortality. Diagnosis of the disease is usually confirmed by the sweat test and duodenal intubation. In children the mean concentration of sodium and chloride ions in the sweat is 20 mmol/l, but in adults this rises to 35 mmol/l. It is accepted that readings above 70 mmol/l indicate the presence of cystic fibrosis.

Measurement of the levels of enzymes in the duodenal juices may also be carried out. The lack of trypsin may indicate the presence of the disease.

The chest radiograph

The chest radiograph may show the effects of airways obstruction due to the lung becoming emphysematous. The diaphragm is flattened and the heart appears narrow. Patchy nodules of consolidation are seen throughout the lung which become more extensive as the disease develops. Thickened and prominent bronchi may also be seen as parallel lines radiating away from the hila.

Treatment and management

The disease is managed with extensive physiotherapy. Postural drainage is widely used. The patient is placed in a head-down position and encouraged to cough. Gravity aids in draining the lung. This is usually carried out at an appointed time every day.

The effects of the disease are treated with antibiotics. The chest infection is treated by using antistaphylococcal antibiotics. These are often routinely given for the first two years of life. Bronchodilators may also be used, particularly if the child develops asthma.

Diet may also be controlled. Steatorrhea is associated with cystic fibrosis and therefore a low fat diet is given. Pancreatic supplements are also given before meals. The overall diet is usually very plain.

Counselling

There is no reliable in utero test for cystic fibrosis. Mothers who have given birth to children with cystic fibrosis have a one in four chance of another child being born with the disease. Unaffected siblings have a one in two chance of carrying the disease. Therefore careful genetic counselling and family support is given.

Patients are now surviving into their fourth decade due to the widespread use of antibiotics and physiotherapy. However, support to the family and patient must be given to help cope with this disabling disease.

Bronchial asthma

Bronchial asthma is a common disease characterized by breathlessness due to generalized narrowing of the airways throughout the lung. It may be subdivided into two types:

(1) Extrinsic asthma. Patients who suffer from this type of asthma can be shown to have an external factor related to their condition that induces the asthma attack. This external factor or allergen may be pollen, dust, etc. and is isolated by carrying out a skin-prick test whereby a number of possible causes for the asthma are introduced under the skin of the patient and the allergic reaction noted.

(2) Intrinsic asthma. The external factor cannot be located in this type of asthma.

Asthma appears in a variety of ways:

(1) Episodic. Here, the asthma attack occurs at any time and is of variable length and severity. The patient wheezes on breathing and complains of a tightness in the chest. Expiration is difficult and breathing is shallow and gasping. A dry cough may also accompany the attack.
(2) Chronic. The patient has a persistent wheeze and cough and is constantly breathless. Chest infections are also common.
(3) Status asthmaticus. This condition is often called severe acute asthma and is classed as an attack of asthma that lasts for more than twenty-four hours and does not respond to medication. The patient develops a tachycardia and in the most advanced cases loses consciousness.

The chest radiograph

The chest radiograph appears normal in all but very advanced cases of asthma. The radiograph is used to show the presence of other conditions that may complicate the treatment, e.g. an underlying pneumonia or pneumothorax.

Treatment

Treatment of asthma involves an attempt to identify any allergens that are prompting the attacks.

Relief and control of asthma

The use of bronchodilators is now widespread. These are usually only given when the disease has been brought under control and other causative factors have been isolated. The bronchodilators help relieve the symptoms of asthma.

The most widely used drug is Salbutamol (Ventolin). This is given in the form of an aerosol spray. The drug is inhaled as a series of puffs, usually up to 3–4 times per day.

Bronchodilators may also be given via a nebulizer. A reservoir containing the solution of bronchodilator is attached to a face mask. Air or oxygen is perfused through the solution which is then inhaled by the patient. Nebulizers deliver a higher dose of drug to the patient and are used in the treatment of chronic asthma. Nebulizers may be used to deliver other drugs such as antibiotics.

Oral or aerosol steroids may also be given to control chronic forms of asthma.

Sarcoidosis

The cause of sarcoidosis is still unknown. The disease manifests itself as widespread areas of granulation tissue. These sarcoid granulomas bear a resemblance to tuberculous lesions prompting a comparison of the two diseases. The sarcoid lesions are widespread and affect many areas of the body.

Areas of involvement

Subcutaneous tissues

Involvement of the subcutaneous tissue produces erythema nodosum. When this occurs it is frequently associated with hilar node enlargement in the chest (see below).

Lymph nodes

These are also frequently involved.

Bones

Bones are rarely affected. If the sarcoid lesion occurs in bone it produces areas of osteoporosis and is largely confined to the feet and hands.

Lungs

This is the commonest site affected by sarcoidosis. The disease produces enlargement of the hilar and paratracheal lymph nodes. This effect is usually bilateral and produces appearances similar to lymphoma. The two may be differentiated by the symmetry of hilar enlargement which is associated with sarcoidosis.

The disease may also show as widespread nodular shadows that have a similar appearance to miliary tuberculosis in advanced cases. Widespread microscopic granuloma are frequently found in cases where bilateral hilar node enlargement is found.

Advanced stages may show a coarse thickening of the lung which indicates a fibrosis of the lung tissue.

Sarcoidosis also affects the eyes, liver, kidneys, skin, central nervous system and spleen.

The Kveim test

This test is carried out to confirm the diagnosis of sarcoidosis. An extract of human sarcoid spleen is injected into the skin. Six weeks later the site is biopsied and the biopsy tested for the presence of sarcoid granuloma. This has a high success rate in diagnosing sarcoidosis.

Treatment

A high proportion of patients with sarcoidosis require no treatment. They usually have no symptoms. Often the enlarged lymph nodes resolve and do not progress to advanced stages.

Treatment may be given if fibrosis develops in the chest or the patient develops symptoms associated with the chest. In this case oral steroids will be given. Steroid treatment may also be given where the eyes and CNS become involved.

Occupational lung diseases

The pneumoconioses

This is a group of diseases that all result from exposure to various forms of dust and particles.

Coalworker's pneumoconiosis (CWP)

This develops as a direct result of prolonged exposure to coal dust. Strenuous efforts are now made to reduce the amount of dust inhaled by coal miners.

The condition is subdivided into a simple pneumoconiosis and a more advanced type called progressive massive fibrosis (PMF).

In simple pneumoconiosis the chest radiograph shows small diffuse coal particles spread throughout the lungs. The patient shows few or no symptoms.

Simple pneumoconiosis has been subdivided into a number of types, dependent upon the extent and appearance of the disease. Thus a standard series of chest radiographs have been prepared to illustrate the types of pneumoconiosis. These standard radiographs help clinicians gauge the extent of the disease.

Treatment. There is no specific treatment for CWP. All patients who have signs of CWP are removed from areas where there is a risk of further exposure to coal dust. This prevents development of PMF.

As PMF progresses it becomes complicated with chronic bronchitis and COAD which then require urgent treatment. Oxygen therapy, steroids and bronchodilators may be given to alleviate the symptoms.

Due to the nature of coalworker's pneumoconiosis and the effect it has on the livelihood of the patient, the extent and control of the disease must be carefully assessed.

Asbestosis

Asbestosis is the result of the inhalation of asbestos dust. It is a form of pneumoconiosis and occurs after occupational exposure to asbestos. Short-term exposure to asbestos is sufficient to produce visible changes on chest radiographs. However, these changes may not be visible until some years after exposure. A more conscious effort is now being made in dealing with asbestos that will reduce the incidence of asbestosis.

Diagnosis

The condition may be diagnosed by characteristic changes seen on the chest radiograph:

(1) Pleural thickening and calcification. Localized areas of pleural thickening and calcification are seen on the lateral aspect of the chest wall. These regions of calcification are harmless, but are useful in indicating the presence of asbestosis.
(2) Diffuse fibrosis. Diffuse areas of fibrous tissue formation may be seen as mottling and streaking throughout the lung.

The patient presents in the early stages with a cough. Asbestos bodies may be present in the sputum. These are pieces of asbestos surrounded by a protein coat. Their presence indicates ingestion of asbestos. As the disease progresses the patient becomes very cyanosed and has increasing difficulty in breathing. Respiratory failure may also develop.

Treatment

Treatment of asbestosis consists of, as with other forms of pneumoconiosis, management of the symptoms that the disease produces. Thus treatment with oxygen therapy, bronchodilators and some steroids is used to alleviate respiratory failure and the bronchitis that may develop.

Complications

(1) Bronchial carcinoma. A large proportion of people occupationally exposed to asbestosis develop bronchial carcinoma.
(2) Mesothelioma. This is a malignant tumour of the pleura that develops many years after exposure to asbestos. The mesothelioma develops out of an area of pleural thickening.

Pneumothorax

When air enters the pleural space the lung collapses. The resulting collapse is called a pneumothorax (Figure 2.7) (Plate 2).

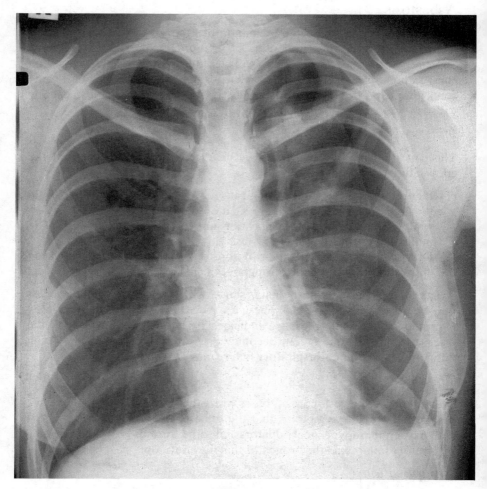

Plate 2   Large pneumothorax of the left lung

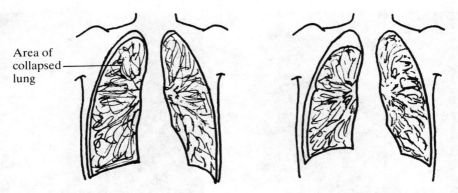

Area of collapsed lung

Figure 2.7 Pneumothorax radiographic appearances: inspiration (left) and expiration (right)

Types

Spontaneous

This type of pneumothorax commonly occurs in young, fit, healthy males. This develops from a leak of air through the apex of the lung. The patient complains of severe, one-sided chest pain of rapid onset. The chest radiograph shows loss of lung markings on the affected side.

Tension

Tension pneumothorax (Figure 2.8) (Plate 3) is a more acute condition than a spontaneous pneumothorax. In this type of pneumothorax, injury to the chest wall produces a 'valve' that allows air into the pleural space on inspiration but closes on expiration and restricts the release of air. This causes a rapid build-up of air in the pleural space. The lung collapses, appears irregularly shaped, and may become compressed to less than half of its expanded size.

The rapid build-up of pressure in the pleura pushes the mediastinum towards the unaffected lung. This may impede expansion of the unaffected lung and cause restriction to blood flow. A tension pneumothorax is diagnosed from a chest radiograph by detecting mediastinal shift.

Tension pneumothorax is classed as an emergency and requires rapid attention.

Treatment

A spontaneous pneumothorax, if small, will generally resolve without being treated. If they do not resolve then the air trapped within the pleural

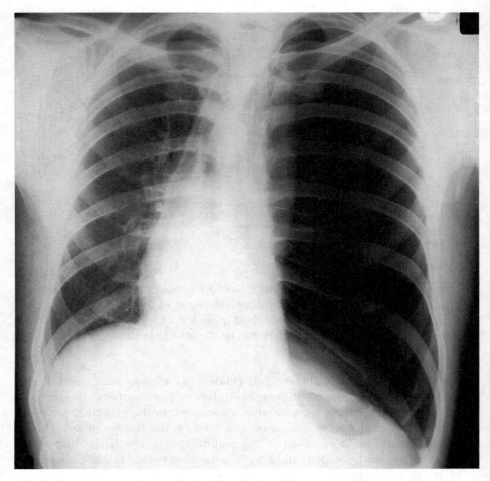

Plate 3   Tension pneumothorax of the left lung. Note movement of the
          mediastinum

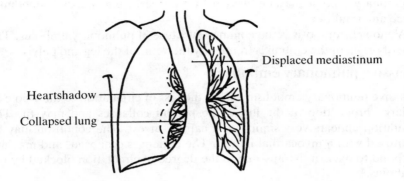

Figure 2.8 Tension pneumothorax showing displacement of the mediastinum to the left

space may be aspirated using a fine needle and syringe. Recurrence of spontaneous pneumothorax may require surgical treatment. A pleurodesis is carried out whereby the pleura is surgically stripped from the chest wall. This causes the build-up of fibrous tissue in the pleural space. The space is eventually obliterated and this prevents any further pneumothorax by sealing the area of leakage.

Tension pneumothorax is corrected by insertion of a catheter into the pleural space. This may be inserted into the axilla or into the anterior chest wall at the level of the third intercostal space. The catheter end is placed underwater in a large bell jar. As the patient breathes air bubbles from the pleural space pass into the water. The bubbling usually stops after twenty-four hours.

Hydropneumothorax

Most cases of pneumothorax are associated with fluid in the pleural cavity. This is usually small and is clearly seen as an air-fluid level on an erect chest radiograph. Pus may be associated with a pneumothorax due to the presence of bacteria in the chest. This is called a pyopneumothorax. If the pneumothorax is associated with an injury to the chest, then the condition is called a haemopneumothorax. Traumatic injury to the chest producing rib fractures may result in a haemopneumothorax.

Pulmonary embolism and infarction

Pulmonary embolism may prove fatal but can be treated. The prognosis depends upon the size and point at which the embolus lodges in the chest.

Pulmonary emboli may be classed by their size, e.g. massive, medium-sized and small.

Venous thrombosis is the commonest cause of pulmonary embolus. The site of origin of the emboli is frequently the veins of the leg and pelvis.

Massive pulmonary embolism

Massive pulmonary embolism causes the loss of circulation to the whole or a large proportion of the lung. The patient collapses and may fit. The condition appears very similar to a cardiac arrest. The condition may be confused with a myocardial infarct. The patient is cyanosed, and may not respond to oxygen therapy due to the degree of circulation blocked by the embolus.

Improvement may be due to movement of the embolus into the lung. If the patient survives the early stages of the attack then there is generally a good prognosis. The extent of the pulmonary infarction may be determined by angiography if the condition of the patient permits.

Medium-sized and small emboli

With small and medium-sized emboli, the condition is not as critical. The patient presents with chest pain and breathlessness. Repeated small emboli occurring over a few months will produce pulmonary hypertension. This is characterized by breathlessness and dyspnoea. This will be seen on the chest radiograph as enlargement of the pulmonary vessels and right ventricle.

If a large embolus is thought to be present in the lung then the chest radiograph may show a raised diaphragm and pleural effusion.

The extent of the infarction is determined by pulmonary angiography and by radionuclide scans. The scan is achieved by (1) injecting albumin labelled with technetium-99m (perfusion scan) or (2) by inhaling radio-labelled xenon. Generally, areas that appear undiseased on chest radiographs but do not take up the isotope are taken as areas affected by pulmonary embolus. This technique may also be used to image for bronchiectasis and emphysema.

Small- or medium-sized pulmonary emboli are treated by the long-term use of anticoagulant therapy.

Respiratory distress syndrome (hyaline membrane disease)

This is one of the most widespread respiratory diseases affecting the new-born. It is commonly found in premature babies (Figure 2.9). The disease is thought to be related to fetal distress in utero and to the lack of

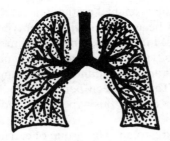

Figure 2.9 Diagrammatic representation of respiratory distress syndrome (hyaline membrane disease)

surfactants at birth. These are chemicals that produce the normal expansion of lung tissue. Lack of surfactants produces solid unexpanded lungs that are unable to carry out gas exchange.

The chest radiograph shows widespread small opacities throughout the lung with the presence of air bronchograms. The bronchi appear visible against the consolidated lung tissue. In advanced cases the lungs appear almost solid.

Adult respiratory distress syndrome (ARDS)

This is a condition that occasionally appears in adults. The lung appears dense and fluid-filled, giving similar appearances to that found in the neonate lung. This condition usually occurs following severe injury to the lung. Trauma to the lung following a car accident or widespread acute infections produce 'shock lung'. This then develops into adult respiratory distress syndrome (ARDS). Excess oxygen and fat embolism are also thought to cause ARDS.

Carcinoma of the bronchus

The incidence of carcinoma of the bronchus is increasing. Smoking is the largest single cause for carcinoma of the bronchus. Other causes include exposure of the patient to chemicals, e.g. cobalt, radioactive substances, atmospheric pollution. It is the commonest primary malignant tumour in the body.

Cell types

Carcinoma of the bronchus is subdivided into four main cell types:

(1) Squamous cell carcinoma. This is found in 35–40 per cent of all cases. This arises through metaplasia (increased rapid growth) of the

squamous cells of the bronchial epithelium. The cells are irregular and this type of cell may be associated with other types of lung cancers.

(2) Oat cell carcinoma. Fifteen per cent of all tumours removed from the bronchus are of this type. Oat cells are closely packed and may secrete hormones. Oat cells are often found in other lung cancers.

(3) Adenocarcinoma. Ten to fifteen per cent of all carcinomas removed from the bronchus are of this type. This type of adenocarcinoma secretes mucus.

(4) Undifferentiated carcinoma. This group of carcinomas is thought to be made up from undifferentiated squamous cell carcinomas and adeno-carcinomas. The cells are large and polygonal. They account for 30 per cent of all tumours of the bronchus.

Tumours of the bronchus may more simply be divided into small and non-small carcinomas.

Site of origin

Most bronchial carcinomas develop in relation to the main bronchi.

Spread

Carcinomas of the bronchus grow quickly and spread by:

(1) Direct invasion. The tumour spreads by direct invasion of surrounding structures. The heart and mediastinum are commonly invaded. The chest wall and pleura may also be involved. Pancoast's tumour involves the brachial plexus and vertebrae. This is an aggressive tumour and causes widespread damage to nerves and other structures in the axilla.

(2) Lymphatic. Invasion of surrounding lymph nodes is also common. Spread is into the hilar nodes. From here the carcinoma may spread to the cervical nodes, axillary nodes, etc. The pulmonary lymphatics may become extensively blocked by cancer cells causing lymphangitis carcinomatosa. This gives rise to widespread oedema of the lung tissue.

(3) Metastatic. Blood-borne metastases are common. Secondary spread is usually to the brain, liver and bones.

Diagnosis

The patient usually presents with a cough, some haemoptysis and hoarseness of the voice. Hoarseness develops due to involvement of the recurrent laryngeal nerve which has a close relationship to the bronchus. A variety of investigations are carried out including bronchoscopy which indicates the extent of any invasion of the bronchus. Biopsy is important in order to classify the cell type present.

The chest radiograph

The cell type cannot be determined from the chest radiograph.

The appearances of carcinoma of the bronchus vary widely depending upon the size and extent of the tumour.

The central mass of the tumour may present as a large hilar mass involving the bronchus. The bronchi may appear narrowed and blunted.

Other effects of the tumour that may also be noted on the chest radiograph are:

(1) There may be involvement of the hilar and mediastinal lymph nodes that will show as enlarged centralized masses.
(2) Involvement of ribs. The ribs may be destroyed by metastatic deposits.
(3) Elevation of the diaphragm.
(4) Pleural effusion and involvement of the chest wall.

Treatment

CT of the chest is often used to show the extent and position of the tumour. Treatment of carcinoma of the bronchus ranges from surgery to chemotherapy. The type of treatment depends upon the extent of the disease:

(1) Palliative treatment. This is given to help relieve symptoms. Palliative surgery may be carried out to remove destructive lesions, e.g. Pancoast's tumour. Palliative radiotherapy may also be used to relieve obstruction and compression of organs and vessels.
(2) Radical treatment. Radical surgery involving the removal of a lobe or lobes together with radical radiotherapy may be carried out to remove and arrest the growth of the tumour.
(3) Chemotherapy. Chemotherapy is often given to treat the tumour and its effects. A regime including vincristine and cyclophosphamide may be used.

Prognosis

The prognosis for untreated cases of carcinoma of the bronchus is poor. Surgical treatment gives a 25–30 per cent five-year survival rate.

Mesothelioma

See asbestosis.

Mediastinal masses

The commonest cause of an underlying mass in the mediastinum is tumour involvement of the lymph nodes (Figure 2.10): Malignant lymphomas commonly show involvement of the mediastinal and hilar lymph nodes.

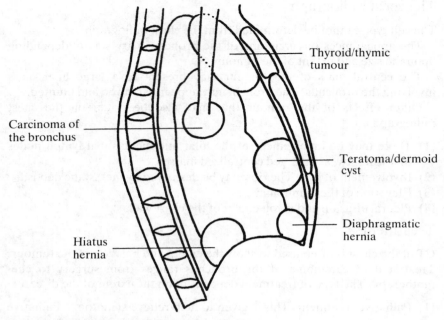

Thyroid/thymic tumour

Carcinoma of the bronchus

Teratoma/dermoid cyst

Diaphragmatic hernia

Hiatus hernia

Figure 2.10 Position of masses within the chest

The pleura

Transudates

This is a non-inflammatory collection of fluid in the pleural cavity (Figure 2.11) and may be associated with pulmonary oedema. If large volumes of transudates build up, then areas of the lung may collapse and cause dyspnoea. Removal of the fluid may be necessary.

Exudates

Exudates all have an underlying iflammatory condition, e.g. pneumonia. The fluid builds up rapidly and may contain organisms related to the underlying cause.

Empyema

This describes the condition of pus in the pleural cavity. This may be due to subphrenic abscess or other lung abscesses. Empyema may be treated by chest drainage and the use of antibiotics. All types of pleural effusion appear the same on chest radiographs. The effusions usually occur between the lobes and at the costophrenic angles.

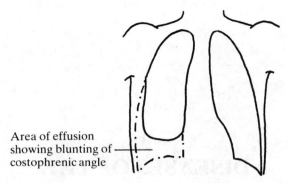

Area of effusion
showing blunting of
costophrenic angle

Figure 2.11 Pleural effusion

Pleural thickening (fibrosis)

Thickening of the pleura may be seen on a chest radiograph following resolution of a pleural effusion. Pleural thickening with calcification is commonly associated with exposure to asbestosis.

Pleural tumours

These are usually metastatic in origin. Mesotheliomas are rare. (See also asbestosis.)

3
DISEASES OF THE
CARDIOVASCULAR SYSTEM

When viewing a chest radiograph taken in the true PA position, the following outline of the heart can be seen (Figure 3.1a).

The right heart border consists of three elements. The most superior portion is the superior vena cava. Below this lies the ascending aorta and the right atrium. The left heart border is made up from the aortic arch, the pulmonary artery, left atrial appendage and the left ventricle.

In the lateral projection (Figure 3.1b) the anterior border of the heart is formed from the pulmonary artery and right ventricle. The posterior border is composed of the left atrium and left ventricle.

Figure 3.2a shows the appearance of the right side of the heart following injection into the superior vena cava. The contrast medium can now be seen to outline the superior vena cava (SVC), the pulmonary artery, right atrium and right ventricle.

Figure 3.2b shows the appearance of the left side of the heart after injection of contrast medium into the left atrium. The contrast medium has clearly outlined the aortic arch, the pulmonary veins by retrograde flow, the left atrium and the left ventricle.

MEASUREMENT OF HEART SIZE

There are a number of methods used to measure the heart size (Figure 3.3). The most commonly used method is to express heart size as the cardiothoracic ratio (CTR). When calculating the cardiothoracic ratio the maximum diameter of the heart (x) is divided by the maximum internal

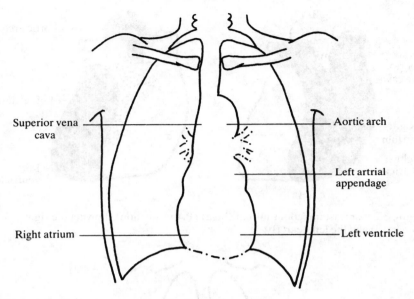

Figure 3.1a Outline of the heart in a PA chest radiograph

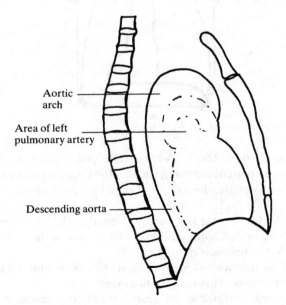

Figure 3.1b Outline of the heart in the left lateral position

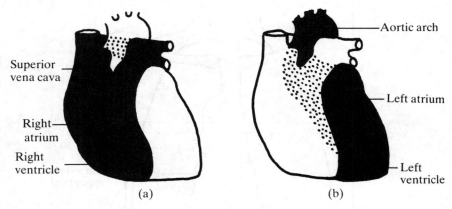

Figure 3.2 Contrast injections into the heart (PA projection) showing the right heart (a) and the left heart (b)

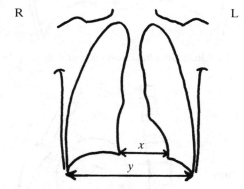

Figure 3.3 The cardiothoracic ratio x/y

diameter of the chest (y) (on a PA chest radiograph taken at 180 cm). It is important that the patient is symmetrical. This ratio is usually less than 0.5 in the majority of people. This method may also be used when measuring heart size in children.

Some radiologists prefer to simply measure the transverse cardiac diameter. In the average adult male this measures less than 15.5 cm and in the average adult female less than 15 cm.

The most accurate measurement of heart size is obtained by comparing the current radiograph to previous radiographs.

The overall shape and size of the heart is often not an accurate indication of heart disease. Heart shape varies considerably. The enlargement of a single heart chamber often cannot be isolated when viewing the chest radiograph as a whole.

THE NORMAL ELECTROCARDIOGRAM

The electrocardiogram (ECG) is obtained by recording tracings from up to twelve leads attached to the chest wall. 'Lead' refers to the ECG obtained as a result of recording the difference in potential between a pair of electrodes. The leads attached to the limbs are called the bipolar or standard leads. The trace is recorded on calibrated graph paper and shows a series of deflections from a baseline. The deflections are designated P, Q, R, S, T and U and the interval between each deflection is called a segment (Figures 3.4a, 3.4b). Thus we have PR, QRS and QT segments.

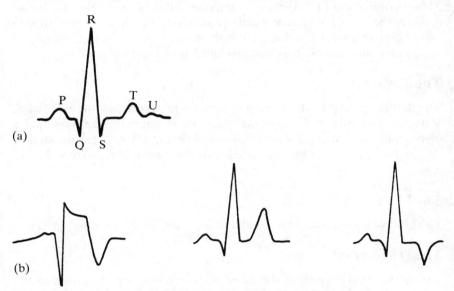

Figure 3.4 ECG normal PQRST complex (a) and abnormal ECG traces (b)

The P wave

The normal P wave is a record of the spread of electrical activity from the sino-atrial node (situated close to the junction of the right atria and superior vena cava) across the atria. The height of the deflection and the duration of the P wave are directly measured from the graph paper on which the ECG is recorded. If the P wave is absent or ectopically placed, this may indicate a block in conduction of electrical impluse to the sino-atrial node.

The PR interval

This corresponds to the time taken for the impulse to travel from the sino-atrial node to the ventricular muscle. On the ECG this is measured from the beginning of the P wave to the beginning of the QRS complex. As the heart rate increases the PR interval decreases, although the lower limit is set at 0.10 second. Below this point the PR interval is classed as abnormal.

The QRS complex

This portion of the ECG represents depolarization of the ventricles. It also involves the spread of electrical activity across the ventricles. Very broad Q waves are often seen associated with myocardial infarct. Generalized ventricular enlargement may also produce a broad QRS complex.

The T wave

The T wave is due to the repolarization, or relaxation, of the ventricles. Very tall and spiked T waves may be seen in patients who have had a myocardial infarction. T wave inversion, where the T wave features below the baseline, may also be associated with the myocardial infarcts (Figure 3.4b).

The U wave

The U wave is not fully understood, but is present in most normal ECGs.

The QT interval

This is the total time from the onset of ventricular depolarization to the completion of repolarization. It is measured from the beginning of the Q wave to the end of the T wave. Prolonged QT intervals are usually associated with the risk of ventricular tachycardia. Decreased QT intervals are associated with an increase in heart rate.

The ST segment

The ST segment lies between the end of the QRS complex and the beginning of the T wave. The ST segment represents a period of constant polarity in the ventricles. The ST segment of the ECG is very useful in diagnosing heart disease. The normal ST segment is situated on the iso-electric line and curves slightly upward.

In acute myocardial infarct the ST segment becomes very elevated. As the episode of myocardial infarction continues, the T wave inverts.

Depression of the ST segment may occur in conditions such as ventricular hypertrophy.

CONGENITAL HEART DISEASE

Congenital heart disease accounts for approximately 10 per cent of all heart conditions found in children. Unless corrected, some congenital heart conditions may shorten the child's expected life-span.

As the embryo develops in utero it undergoes radical changes. The heart is first formed as a simple tube. As the embryo grows this subdivides into five segments (Figure 3.5) from which the four-chambered vessel of the heart forms. Between the fifth and eighth weeks of embryonic develop-ment the greatest changes to the heart take place. These include subdivision of the chambers by septal formation. By the end of the eighth week the heart has assumed the appearance of the complete adult heart.

The right atrium of the fetal circulation receives blood from the SVC and vitello-umbilical veins which later form the inferior vena cava (IVC). Some of the venous blood passes into the right IVC ventricle and then on to the pulmonary artery. This blood eventually reaches the aorta by way of the

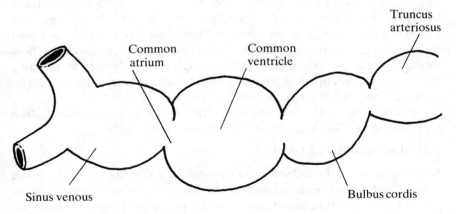

Figure 3.5 The rudimentary heart

ductus arteriosus. It is during this period of rapid growth that most malformations develop.

The causes of congenital heart disease are little understood. Often no cause can be found for a child born with a congenital abnormality of the heart. A small proportion can be clearly linked to genetic problems. Twenty per cent of children with congenital heart disease show congenital abnormalities in other organs, e.g. Down's Syndrome. Other factors are more clearly linked to the production of abnormalities:

(1) Viral infections. If the mother contracts rubella virus (German measles) within the first three months of pregnancy, then there is increased risk of congenital abnormalities affecting the heart, eyes and brain.
(2) Syphilis and the vitamin deficiency diseases.

Disorders of the whole heart

Dextrocardia

Complete mirror image of the heart together with the viscera occurs once in every 5,000 births. This usually does not lead to any medical problems. An incomplete condition is also found involving either (1) reversed heart position and normal viscera or (2) normal heart position and reversed viscera. These conditions usually cause complications and require surgical correction.

Defects of the septum

The pressures in the normal heart, when measured via catheterization, are found to be lower on the right than on the left. When the two communicate, as with some abnormalities, there is a shunt of blood through the defect from left to right. This results in an increased blood flow through the lungs. This increased blood flow causes damage to the lung tissue and a consequent increase in pulmonary vascular resistance. The resistance may increase to cause eventually a reverse shunt.

Defects between the left and right sides of the heart are called atrial septal defects (ASD) and ventricular septal defects (VSD).

Atrial septal defect (ASD)

In the fetus the right and left atria communicate directly via the foramen ovale. The foramen ovale normally closes shortly after birth. It may remain patent but generally does not allow blood flow across the atrial septum because of its valve-like structure (Figure 3.6). However, there are two main

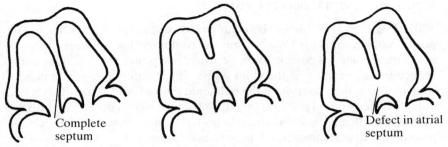

Figure 3.6 Atrial septal defect (ASD): unaffected heart (left); ostium primum (middle) and ostium secundum (right)

types of abnormality that do permit blood flow across:

(1) Ostium secundum. This type of defect involves the lower part of the atrial septum.
(2) Ostium primum. This is the commonest and most easily corrected type. The opening is of variable size and site and does not involve the atrioventricular valves (mitral and tricuspid valves).

The defect may also extend caudally to involve the atrioventricular valves. The ventricular septum may also be affected. Corrective surgery may be performed by fixing a patch over the opening. The patch usually consists of man-made fibres, e.g. Dacron.

In cases of ASD blood flow becomes preferential through the right ventricle due to the lower right heart pressure. Blood flow through the pulmonary circulation is usually two to three times higher than the aortic blood flow. This will cause enlargement and hypertrophy of the right ventricle (RV) and eventual damage to the lungs from pulmonary hypertensions. Defects are detected by ECG changes.

The chest radiograph shows an enlarged heart with prominent pulmonary vessels. The aorta appears much smaller than normal. Echocardiography can be used to localize the defect and to differentiate between primary and secondary defects.

Cardiac catheterization may also be used to show the extent and position of the defect prior to surgery. An injection of contrast medium is given into the upper right pulmonary vein and cine films are taken in an oblique projection to profile the atrial septum. Contrast medium may also be injected into the left ventricle if the catheter tip is passed through the atrial wall. Oxygen saturation levels are also taken at the time of catheterization.

Radionuclide scans may also be carried out to measure the extent of the shunt from left to right.

Ventricular septal defect (VSD)

VSD (Figure 3.7) is one of the commonest congenital heart lesions. The position of the defect is variable, but the commonest site is near the aorta in the membraneous portion of the ventricular septum. Small VSDs usually reduce in size or close as the child grows. If the defect remains, and is of sufficient size, then damage to the pulmonary vessels will result. This is due to high velocity blood passing from the left ventricle on contraction into the right ventricle and out into the lungs. This may result in irreversible pulmonary hypertension, and in this case surgery to close the VSD is contraindicated.

If the resistance of the pulmonary vessels has remained low then the volume of blood from left to the right increases.

Large left to right shunts are liable to produce cardiac failure in the second or third months after birth. If a large shunt does not produce symptoms within the first few years, then problems will not develop until the child reaches early adulthood. Symptoms such as fatigue and breathlessness will then be noted.

Large VSDs will produce significant heart murmurs and changes to the ECG. The chest radiograph will also show changes of cardiomegaly with or without pulmonary hypertension when the shunt is large, e.g. 2:1 between the ventricles. The pulmonary artery will appear prominent and the heart will be enlarged. Enlargement of the ventricles will also be seen on echocardiography.

Cardiac catheterization is carried out to determine the position of the VSD. Oxygen saturations are taken in the right ventricle and the left ventricle if the septum can be crossed. Biopsy of the lung tissue may also be

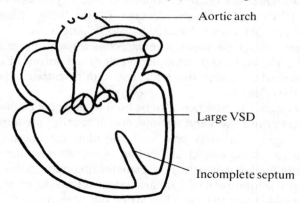

Figure 3.7   Ventricular septal defect (VSD)

taken to show the extent of any damage to the lung tissue. Cine angiography is then carried out by injecting contrast medium into the left ventricle and placing the child in an oblique position to profile the ventricle septum. This is usually achieved by catheterizing the femoral or brachial artery. The left ventricle is entered by catheterizing the femoral or brachial arteries. The femoral vein is also catheterized to measure oxygen saturation in the right heart. The VSD may also be diagnosed by an isotope scan. Large VSDs are surgically closed.

Other congenital heart lesions

Patent ductus arteriosus

In utero, oxygenated blood passes from the pulmonary circulation into the aorta via the ductus arteriosus (Figure 3.8). This usually closes shortly after birth. However, in some children it either partly closes or remains open and allows the passage of high velocity blood from the aorta into the main pulmonary artery, leading to pulmonary hypertension.

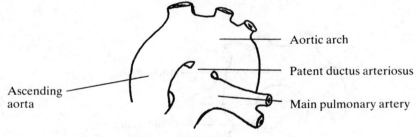

Aortic arch

Patent ductus arteriosus

Ascending aorta

Main pulmonary artery

Figure 3.8 Patent ductus arteriosus (PDA)

Heart failure may also result due to the loss of blood into the pulmonary circulation. Infection of the heart with *Streptococcus viridans* is also associated with patent ductus arteriosus.

The condition is characterized by a continous heart murmur that is due to blood passing through the ductus throughout the cardiac cycle. Other heart murmurs may be heard due to the increased blood return from the lungs to the heart.

If the ductus is large then the left ventricle and left atrium will begin to hypertrophy. This may be seen on the chest radiograph together with enlarged pulmonary vessels and aorta. Cine angiography in the lateral position may be carried out to show the presence of the opening.

The ductus is closed by surgical ligation within the first few years of life.

Coarctation of the aorta

Coarctation of the aorta (Figure 3.9) is narrowing of the lumen of the aorta. This usually occurs just beyond the origin of the left subclavian artery. The condition may be associated with persistence of the ductus arteriosus and a bicuspid aortic valve.

The systolic pressure in the aorta proximal to the coarctation is usually raised. When the coarctation is causing severe narrowing of the aorta, large collateral vessels develop to bypass the narrowing. Hypertension may be associated with the condition.

The femoral arterial pulse is usually feeble and delayed in patients with a severe coarctation and a systolic heart murmur may also be heard. The chest radiograph in children may be normal while in the adult an enlarged aortic knuckle may be seen together with notching of the underside of the ribs. This is due to hypertrophied intercostal collateral arteries in the chest.

The condition may be corrected by surgical removal of the coarctation and anastomosis of the ends. Balloon angioplasty is now being used to dilate the structure.

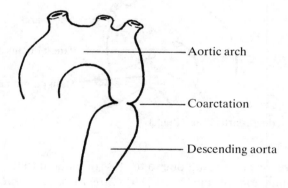

Figure 3.9   Coarctation of the aorta

Abnormalities of the valves

Aortic valve

Aortic valve stenosis may be found in some newborn children. The abnormality may involve the valve or the aorta distal to the valve. Supravalvar aortic stenosis is particularly associated with congenital abnormalities of the heart.

Pulmonary stenosis

Pulmonary stenosis is usually congenital. The pulmonary valve is abnormal, the cusps becoming fused. This causes obstruction to blood flow and a jet develops at the centre of the valve. The area beyond the lesion becomes dilated and the right ventricle becomes hypertrophied. As the right ventricle enlarges the right atrium forcibly contracts to help eject blood from the right side of the heart.

The ECG shows the presence and extent of the pulmonary stenosis. Chest radiographs will show an enlarged heart and dilated pulmonary outflow tract. Cardiac catheterization may be carried out to measure the pressure gradient across the valve. A pressure drop of 50 mmHg is considered as severe stenosis. Cine angiography may be taken in the lateral position to demonstrate valve narrowing. Surgical correction or balloon angioplasty (pulmonary valvotomy) of the valve may be carried out to correct the condition.

Combined congenital heart abnormalities

Fallot's tetralogy

The tetralogy of Fallot (Figure 3.10a) is a combination of the following four conditions that are all present at birth:

(1) Pulmonary stenosis.
(2) A VSD.
(3) Dextraposition of the aorta with overriding of the aorta. The aorta is situated close to the VSD and receives blood from the left and right ventricle.
(4) Right ventricular hypertrophy.

The condition presents as severe breathlessness and cyanosis. Seventy per cent of children exhibiting cyanosis on investigation are found to have the tetralogy.

The chest radiograph (Figure 3.10b) is very characteristic as the heart becomes 'boot-shaped' due to right ventricular hypertrophy.

Echocardiography will show the extent of the abnormalities and generally cine angiography is not required. Cardiac catheterization will show:

(1) Similar pressures in the right and left ventricles.
(2) A pressure drop between the body of the right ventricle and the outflow tract.
(3) Oxygen saturations in the aorta are abnormally low.

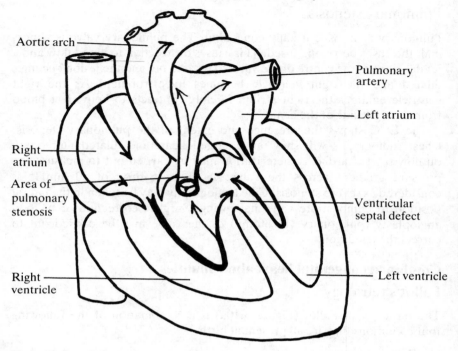

Figure 3.10a Fallot's tetralogy

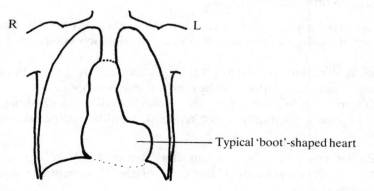

Figure 3.10b Appearance of Fallot's heart on a PA chest radiograph

Injection of contrast into the right ventricle shows the region of pulmonary stenosis and the VSD.

The tetralogy must be surgically corrected. If left uncorrected, death will result from cerebrovascular accidents or infective problems (e.g. sub-acute bacterial endocarditis). Surgery is carried out mainly by two methods:

(1) Waterston operation. In this operation a direct shunt is created between the aorta and the pulmonary circulation.
(2) Blalock-Taussig procedure. This creates a similar shunt between the right subclavian artery and the right pulmonary artery.

Both methods will allow an increased blood flow through the lungs thus allowing more blood to become oxygenated.

Displacement of vessels

Transposition of the great vessels

In transposition of the great vessels, the aorta arises from the right ventricle and the pulmonary artery from the left ventricle. The condition is usually accompanied by another heart defect, e.g. ASD, VSD. This malformation allows mixing of deoxygenated and oxygenated blood within the heart. Echocardiography may be used to demonstrate the position of the vessels. Cardiac angiography may also be required.

The condition must be quickly corrected within the first few weeks of life. If the newborn child is acutely ill, then a deliberate hole may be created in the heart. This is done by passing a deflated balloon catheter through the atrial septum via the existing foramen ovale. The balloon catheter is then inflated and pulled back through the septum, from RA to LA. This tears the septum and gives mixing of the systemic and pulmonary blood. This is called the Rashkind procedure and can be carried out on the premature baby unit under ultrasound control. This will sustain the child through the initial neonatal period. Surgical correction is then carried out.

ACQUIRED HEART DISEASE

Diseases of the coronary ateries

The coronary circulation

The right and left coronary arteries comprise the coronary circulation (Figure 3.11).

The right coronary artery arises in the right coronary sinus of Valsalva

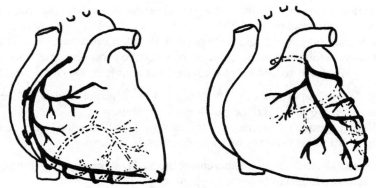

Figure 3.11   Coronary circulation of the right coronary artery (left) and the left coronary artery (right)

and runs between the right ventricle and right atrium. The right coronary supplies the atrioventricular node, the sinus node, right ventricle and posterior portion of the left ventricle.

The left coronary artery arises in the left coronary sinus of Valsalva and divides into two main branches:

(1) The left anterior descending branch (LAD). This branch runs anteriorly between the two ventricles and supplies the interventricular septum and the anterior wall of the left ventricle.
(2) The left circumflex branch. This branch passes down between the left atrium and left ventricle and supplies the lateral and posterior aspects of the left ventricle.

The left coronary artery eventually drains into the coronary sinus while the right coronary artery drains into the cardiac veins. Both then drain into the right atrium.

The coronary circulation differs from other regions in that the coronary arteries fill only during diastole. This is due to the myocardium compressing the coronary arteries in systole, preventing blood flow.

Coronary artery disease

Coronary artery disease is the commonest cause of heart disease and is primarily caused by atherosclerosis, which describes a number of changes that take place in the walls of arteries. The changes include deposition on the intima of lipids, blood, fibrous tissue and calcium. The resulting deposited products form a plaque on the arterial wall. Advanced plaques may become necrotic at their centres. The plaque may continue to grow and block off the vessel, or break up and cause further distal emboli.

The mechanism for the build-up of the coronary atherosclerosis is thought to be due to lipid infiltration, the theory of which proposes that some plasma products, especially lipids, infiltrate through the wall of the artery. The presence of the lipids promotes the proliferation of smooth muscle which leads to the formation of atherosclerosis.

This theory is supported by the fact that people with high lipid plasma levels show an increased incidence of atherosclerotic heart disease. A high lipid plasma level is a familial trait that is called hyperlipoproteinaemia. Groups that show the greatest risk tend to have increased levels of cholesterol in their blood. Smoking and diabetes mellitus also increase the risk of heart disease.

The presence of atherosclerosis produces a number of conditions that are classed under the heading of ischaemic heart disease. These include angina pectoris, myocardial infarcts, sudden death and the disruption of normal heart rhythm.

Angina pectoris

Angina pectoris occurs when blood supply to the myocardium is insufficient. The waste products of metabolism, e.g. lactic acid, begin to build up and cause severe pain.

Angina pectoris is most often felt behind the middle or upper part of the sternum. The pain may become very intense and radiate down the arms or up around the jaw. The pain is frequently described as a tight band or heavy weight. Angina attacks are usually prompted by exertion and the pain lasts for usually more than thirty seconds but less than fifteen minutes. The ECG, particularly when taken on exertion, will show depression of the ST segment.

It is difficult to observe and monitor attacks of angina because their occurrence is difficult to predict. Therefore the patient carries out an exercise test. This is conducted in the cardiac department with the patient under close supervision. The patient walks on a treadmill while an ECG is taken. The exercise test is staged and a note made of where the patient first experiences chest pain. The ECG is continued after the exercise has finished to detect resting angina following exercise. The patient may also be examined by carrying out coronary angiography to detect any narrowing or blocks in the arteries.

Angina pectoris is often associated with stress and is exaggerated by smoking. Removing these factors helps control the symptoms. The pain can also be controlled by giving drugs, e.g. glyceryl trinitrate. Further treatment may be given in the form of physiotherapy to build up exercise tolerance. In some cases coronary artery bypass grafts or coronary angioplasty may be carried out.

Myocardial infarction

Myocardial infarction (MI) is the distruction of a portion of the myocardium. This is due to severe and prolonged ischaemia to the heart muscle. Myocardial infarction accounts for approximately 15 per cent of all deaths. It is more common in males than in females.

When an area of the heart becomes ischaemic the small anastomoses that connect the coronary arteries enlarge and form a collateral circulation. The location and extent of the myocardial infarct depends upon the coronary artery that has blocked, and the extent of the collateral circulation.

Occlusion of the circumflex artery causes infarction of the lateral or posterior walls of the left ventricle, while occlusion of the right coronary artery causes infarction of the inferior portion of the left ventricle and the entire right ventricle.

The most common area of occlusion is the left anterior descending segment of the left coronary artery. Most blocks usually occur 2–3 cm beyond the origin of the coronary artery. The infarct affects the anterior wall of the left ventricle and the septum.

Acute myocardial infarction requires immediate medical care. Many patients complain of periods of angina and breathlessness before the attack takes place. The pain occurs in the chest and arms and is not relieved by resting.

Cardiac arrhythmias and heart failure are closely associated with myocardial infarcts and account for 80–90 per cent of all mortalities from MI when they occur together, especially in the first few minutes.

Myocardial infarction is diagnosed by ECG changes. The ECG shows elevation of the ST segment with inversion of the T waves. These changes are thought to be due to damage to the myocardium.

The increased presence of certain enzymes in the blood serum may also indicate the presence and extent of a myocardial infarct. One example is serum creatine phosphokinase. This is present in the myocardium in large amounts following MI. Following a myocardial infarct, the level of this enzyme in the blood plasma rises as a result of necrosis of the myocardium.

The condition is treated in its early stages by giving drugs to relieve chest pain. Strong analgesics such as diamorphine or intravenous morphine sulphate are given together with oxygen. The patient is then admitted to intensive care or onto the coronary care unit to be closely observed and monitored.

Chest radiographs are of little value in the early stages of myocardial infarction, particularly if carried out by a mobile X-ray unit. LV and coronary angiography are necessary to demonstrate the extent of the damage to the heart. Chest radiographs are necessary to show pulmonary oedema.

Rheumatic heart disease

Rheumatic fever is an immunological disease that develops following infection by group A – haemolytic streptococci, e.g. *Streptococcus pyogenes*. It is now uncommon.

Ninety per cent of the first attacks of rheumatic fever occur between the ages of 5–15 years. The disease is preceded by a generalized streptococcal infection and fever but the connection between rheumatic fever and streptococcal infections is not clear. If the initial infection is treated with penicillin then rheumatic fever is usually prevented. If not treated the disease occurs periodically and leads to inflammatory changes of connective tissue. There is also involvement of the joints, blood vessels, lungs and, most importantly, the heart:

(1) The joints. The disease (polyarthritis) usually affects the large joints and is similar to rheumatoid arthritis. However, the effect is transient and leaves no permanent disability.
(2) The blood vessels. An acute inflammation of the blood vessels may occur. This is usually widespread and affects the coronary, pulmonary and cerebral arteries.
(3) The brain. About 30 per cent of patients with acute rheumatic fever show signs of cerebral irritation. This may be associated with involuntary, irregular muscle contractions. This is commonly called St Vitus' dance or Sydenham's chorea.
(4) The heart. Chronic rheumatic heart disease affects the pericardium, myocardium and the endocardium.
  (a) Myocardium. The myocardium shows widespread growth of Aschoff nodes. These develop in the atrial and ventricular myocardium. They are composed of a mixture of fibroblasts and lymphocytes and may show areas of necrosis. The presence of Aschoff nodes confirms the diagnosis of rheumatic myocarditis. The scarring produced by the nodes, together with the myocarditis, may lead to death.
  (b) Endocardium. Involvement of the endocardium leads to damage of the heart valves. The mitral valve is the most commonly affected single valve. Disease of the mitral valve in combination

with the aortic valve is also commonly seen. The pulmonary and tricuspid valves are rarely affected.

The affected valves become thickened. The surface of the valves then becomes eroded; vegetations form on the chordae tendinae and at the point at which the valves close. As the disease continues the valves become increasingly thickened and distorted due to the production of fibrous tissue. The valves become stenosed and deformed due to contraction of the chordae tendinae. Later stages may show deposition of calcium in the valves. This may be clearly seen on chest radiography.

Clear diagnosis of rheumatic fever is difficult and is confirmed as a combination of factors such as the presence of a throat infection together with pericarditis and polyarthritis. ECG changes may also be noted such as an increased PR interval.

Chronic rheumatic heart disease ultimately produces extensive valve disease involving stenosis of the valves, regurgitation and valve incompetence (see below).

Treatment and prevention

All patients who develop acute rheumatic fever are treated with doses of penicillin. This may be continued into adulthood to prevent recurrence. Control of chronic rheumatic fever is more difficult. Patients may be given steroids and salicylates to relieve the effects of polyarthritis. However, damage to the heart valves is difficult to control.

Diseases of the cardiac valves

Mitral valve disease

Mitral stenosis

Mitral stenosis is caused by (1) recurrent rheumatic fever and (2) infective endocarditis due to the presence of A-haemolytic streptococci, pneumococci, etc.

The mitral valve leaflets adhere to each other due to the presence of fibrous tissue leaving a central jet. The narrowing causes problems when the mitral valve has narrowed from the normal adult valve of 5 cm² to 1 cm². Narrowing of the valve produces an increase in the pressure gradient across the valve opening. This also produces an increase in pressure of the left atrium and in size. The normal resting pressure in the left atrium is 12 mmHg, but in severe mitral stenosis this rises to 25 mmHg.

A rise in pressure in the left atrium will also cause a pressure rise in the pulmonary veins and capillaries. If the increase in pressure in the pulmonary vessels is rapid, pulmonary oedema will result. This causes the patient acute breathlessness.

Diagnosis. Mitral stenosis shows changes in the echocardiogram, characterized by increase in the height of the P wave and atrial fibrillation.

The chest radiograph will show an increase in the size of the left atrial appendage. Backward displacement of the oesophagus may also be seen during a barium swallow. The lateral view will show posterior enlargement of the atrium. The pulmonary oedema associated with mitral stenosis will also be visible on the chest radiograph. Interstitial oedema develops due to thickening of the septa throughout the lung. The thickened septa produce lines in the lung tissue. In mitral stenosis peripherally thickened septal lines may be seen. These are called Kerley B lines. These radiate laterally in the lower zones and merge into the lung edge. The upper pulmonary vessels may also appear dilated.

Cardiac catheterization may be carried out to measure the gradient across the mitral valve and to screen for aortic valve disease. Mitral stenosis is commonly combined with aortic regurgitation (see below).

Treatment. Mitral stenosis usually requires surgical intervention:

(1) Mitral valvotomy. This may be carried out as an open heart procedure or as closed procedure. The valve may be enlarged by using a balloon catheter. This is usually carried out when the disease is attributable only to mitral stenosis.
(2) Mitral valve replacement. Involving replacement of the mitral valve with a prosthesis.

Mitral regurgitation

The causes of mitral regurgitation or mitral valve incompetence are very similar to those of mitral stenosis – usually rheumatic fever and infective endocarditis. Rheumatic fever commonly causes prolapse of the mitral valve.

Due to the relationship of the aortic valve to the mitral valve, changes in the aortic valve and left ventricle directly affect the mitral valve.

Left ventricular dilation leads to dilatation of the entire valve ring. The disruption to the mitral valve causes mitral regurgitation which causes further enlargement of the left ventricle and retrogradely to the lungs.

Any condition that impedes left ventricle output or causes stenosis of the aortic valve will also produce mitral regurgitation.

As the disease progresses the left ventricle becomes hypertrophied, the left atrium dilates and pulmonary hypertension develops. Severe pulmonary hypertension and right-sided heart failure only develop when mitral stenosis and mitral regurgitation are present together.

The disease is diagnosed from abnormal heart sounds and an abnormal ECG that shows abnormal P waves or atrial fibrillation.

Patients usually present with tiredness and dyspnoea. In cases of acute mitral regurgitation the patient will present with acute pulmonary oedema. Patients with mitral regurgitation will present with acute pulmonary oedema.

The diagnosis is confirmed by carrying out cardiac catheterization. Injecting contrast medium into the left ventricle will demonstrate the extent of the mitral regurgitation. A dilated left ventricle may also be demonstrated.

Patients with mild mitral regurgitation may live a relatively normal life. However, if the disease is complicated by other heart problems then the valve must be corrected. Mitral regurgitation may only successfully be corrected by surgical means. The valve may be repaired but is usually replaced by a prosthesis.

Aortic valve disease

Aortic stenosis

Aortic stenosis (Figure 3.12) usually occurs at the level of the aortic valve or just below the aortic cusps (subvalvar stenosis). Aortic stenosis is caused by:

(1) Congenital malformations. This is frequently subvalvar.
(2) Rheumatism. This is the commonest cause and is associated with thickening and calcification of the aortic cusps. Aortic regurgitation is often related to rheumatic disease of the aortic valve. However,

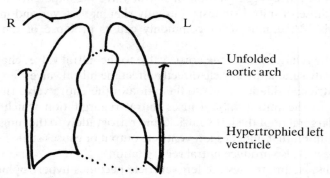

R   L

Unfolded aortic arch

Hypertrophied left ventricle

Figure 3.12   The effects of severe aortic stenosis

stenosis of the mitral valve predominates over that of the aortic valve in cases of rheumatic heart disease.

(3) Calcified aortic stenosis. Calcified arteries and the aortic valve are frequently seen in the elderly. This causes rigidity of the valve and aorta and severe aortic stenosis.

(4) Infection. Endocarditis may also cause aortic stenosis.

Aortic stenosis give rise to an increase in ventricular systolic pressure as the ventricle contracts more forcibly against the stenosis. The left ventricle hypertrophies and becomes less efficient at pumping blood. The left atrium may enlarge. The left ventricle continues to hypertrophy and dilate as not all the cardiac output is ejected. The coronary arteries enlarge to keep pace with increasing demand for blood. The patient suffers from increasing breathlessness and episodes of angina pectoris. Angina is more commonly associated with aortic valve disease than with any other type of valve disease.

The disease is diagnosed via an abnormal pulse and abnormal heart sounds. The ECG will demonstrate left ventricular hypertrophy.

Calcification of the aortic valve may also be seen in patients with rheumatic heart conditions, and in the elderly. In later stages left ventricular enlargement is seen.

Cardiac catheterization is carried out to measure the pressure gradient across the stenosed valve and to check for aortic regurgitation. Possible damage to the coronary arteries is also assessed.

Surgical treatment is carried out in cases of severe aortic stenosis. The valve may be repaired in cases of congenital abnormalities or replaced with a prosthesis if the valve is heavily calcified.

Aortic regurgitation

The causes of aortic regurgitation are the same as for aortic stenosis. Blood passes back into the aorta as a result of damage to the aortic valve and this results in enlargement of the left ventricle to compensate for this backward movement of blood.

The patient presents with breathlessness and angina pectoris. The ECG shows evidence of left ventricular hypertrophy. The chest radiograph shows an enlargement of the left ventricle and dilation of the ascending aorta. Cardiac catheterization is carried out to demonstrate the extent of the regurgitation.

Mild cases of aortic regurgitation require little or no treatment. The patient may simply restrict activity and decrease the demand on the heart. In severe cases surgery may be carried out to replace the aortic valve.

Tricuspid valve disease

Tricuspid valve disease is the least common of any types of valve disease and is almost always caused by rheumatic heart disease. It rarely occurs as an isolated lesion.

Tricuspid stenosis

This is a rare condition. Tricuspid stenosis is commonly associated with mitral stenosis. The patient presents with breathlessness that is usually not as severe as in mitral valve disease. The chest radiograph shows enlargement of the right atrium and SVC. In severe cases the disease is treated by valve replacement.

Tricuspid regurgitation

Tricuspid regurgitation usually occurs together with mitral valve disease. The disease is commonly caused by rheumatic fever. The disease produces right-sided heart problems with right-sided heart failure and venous congestion. Radiographic appearances are similar to those seen in tricuspid stenosis. Cardiac catheterization may be carried out if the regurgitation is thought to be severe. In severe cases tricuspid regurgitation is corrected by surgical replacement of the diseased valve.

Pulmonary valve disease

Pulmonary valve disease is quite uncommon. It is rarely associated with rheumatic heart disease. Pulmonary stenosis is most commonly associated with congenital abnormalities (see p.49). Pulmonary regurgitation is usually associated with other types of heart disease.

Aneurysms

An aneurysm is an abnormal localized dilatation of a vessel or chamber, of which there are two types, true aneurysms and false aneurysms:

True

There are three types (Figure 3.13) of true aneurysm:

(1) Saccular. A small portion of the vessel expands to produce a uniform localized swelling.
(2) Fusiform. Generalized swelling of the vessel over a large area. The overall diameter of the vessel increases and may cause bony erosions.
(3) Dissecting. A false lumen develops within the vessel due to separation of the wall into an inner layer of intima and part of the media, and an

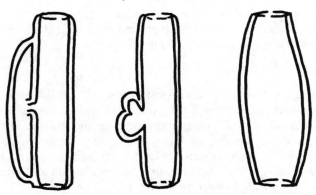

Figure 3.13   Types of aneurysm: dissecting (left); saccular (middle) and fusiform (right)

outer layer of adventitia and the remaining media. Blood may then enter this false lumen.

The following are examples of true aneurysms:

(1) Berry aneurysm. This is a congenitally linked aneurysm that is found intracranially in the circle of Willis. It is particularly common at the junctions of the anterior or posterior communicating arteries. The aneurysm is due to a defect in the arterial wall. As growth takes place the wall becomes more fragile until a saccular aneurysm develops. The patient may complain of pain. Blood in the stained CSF may indicate leakage of the aneurysm. Rupture of the aneurysm produces a sub-arachnoid haemorrhage or rupture of the ventricles.

(2) Arteriovenous malformations (AVM). This is an uncommon congenital abnormality of blood vessels composed of localized groups of poorly formed blood vessels. These may develop in the brain and are called 'angiomas'. They also occur at other sites, e.g. lungs, limbs. Rupture of AVM will cause haemorrhage. Large lesions may be treated by embolisation under screening and angiographic control.

(3) Dissecting aneurysms. These most commonly occur in the aorta due to the breakdown of the media. Blood enters the wall of the artery and tracks between the intima and the adventitia. This produces a false lumen that runs parallel to the vessel. This is clearly seen during angiography. The dissection does not remain localized but travels along the vessel. The dissection may develop slowly and obliterate adjoining vessels. This will cause loss of circulation to other organs. The vessel will usually rupture either into the lumen of the blood vessel

or into the surrounding tissues. External rupture is the most common and causes massive haemorrhage around the site of the leak. External rupture will usually result in rapid death.

False

False aneurysms develop due to perforation of arterial walls, usually following trauma. Blood leaks into the surrounding tissue causing the build-up of haematoma. Blood pressures inside and outside of the vessel stabilize and allow pooling of blood inside the haematoma, and the haematoma will be seen to pulse. The haematoma is removed and the damaged vessel sutured. Communication between a vein and artery within a false aneurysm is called an arteriovenous fistulae.

Cardiomyopathy

Cardiomyopathy describes a group of diseases that all produce abnormalities of the myocardium. This may be due to alcoholic poisoning or through nutritional abnormalities. Cardiomyopathy may also occur in relation to other diseases, e.g. cystic fibrosis, myxoedema and thyrotoxicosis. Cardiomyopathies are difficult to diagnose and frequently require biopsy of the myocardium under fluoroscopic control.

Hypertrophic obstructive cardiomyopathy (HOCM)

HOCM refers to an idiopathic disease which causes outflow tract obstruction on either the left of right side of the heart.

Hypertension

Hypertension is classified as a sustained rise in the systemic blood pressure above 140 mmHg systolic and 90 mmHg diastolic in a resting individual. Hypertension is classed as severe if the diastolic pressure rises above approximately 115 mmHg. There are two types of hypertension:

(1) Primary or essential. If no known cause for the hypertension can be discovered, the hypertension is described as primary. Approximately 90 per cent of patients have this type of hypertension.
(2) Secondary. The hypertension has a readily and sometimes treatable, identifiable cause.

Primary

This category is further subdivided into 'benign' and 'malignant' hypertension.

Benign

This is a common condition in which there is a slow progressive rise in blood pressure over a number of years. The disease accelerates in its latter stages. Benign hypertension produces left ventricular hypertrophy and the build-up of atheroma in arteries. Arteriosclerotic changes take place in small arteries and vascular changes in various organs. Renal failure and cerebrovascular accidents are complications of benign hypertension. Smoking and obesity and heredity factors can be linked to 'benign' hypertension.

Malignant

This condition may follow benign hypertension or it may develop as an isolated condition. Malignant hypertension is characterized by rapid and sustained increase in blood pressure. If untreated the disease is complicated by renal and heart failure and intracranial haemorrhage.

Secondary

Secondary hypertension develops as a result of another disease. The conditions most commonly associated with secondary hypertension are renal disease, brain tumours or haemorrhage and pregnancy.

Renal disease

The role of the kidney in hypertension is related to the levels of renin and angiotensin present in the bloodstream. Both renin and angiotensin have vasoconstrictive effects.

A number of renal conditions cause hypertension. These include:

(1) Polycystic disease of the kidney leading to renal failure.
(2) Narrowing of the renal artery stenosis causes hypertension to develop.
(3) Primary aldosteronism (Conn's syndrome). Over-secretion of aldosterone leads to hypertension.
(4) Phaeochromocytoma. Phaeochromocytomas are found in the adrenal glands. They are mostly benign tumours and secrete noradrenaline or adrenaline which is responsible for the increase in blood pressure.
(5) Cushing's syndrome. Increased production of adrenocorticotrophin (ACTH). Steroid therapy causes hypertension.

Brain

Increased intracranial pressure due to the presence of tumours or haemorrhage may also be responsible for hypertension.

Pregnancy

Hypertension may develop during pregnancy, usually in III trimester. This is usually mild but in some it may become chronic and may require extra treatment. This condition is called pre-eclampsia.

Pulmonary

Normal pulmonary blood flow is 5–8 litre/minute at rest. Normal pulmonary blood pressure is 16–17 mmHg. The pulmonary circulation is designed to withstand large changes in the pulmonary blood flow while maintaining normal pulmonary pressure. The walls of the pulmonary vessels are very elastic and easily carry the pressure loading from the right ventricle. Pulmonary hypertension develops from a number of causes:

(1) Passive. Mitral valve disease may cause the build-up of atheroma and the possibility of formation of emboli.
(2) Increased flow. This is due to:
    (a) ASD left to right shunts. In the end stages the pulmonary resistance is so high as to produce a reverse in the shunt from left to right.
    (b) VSD. In this case the pulmonary vessels come under the full force of the left ventricular pressure from birth. This causes severe damage to the child's lungs and is a more severe condition than ASD.
(3) Organic obstruction.

Loss of pulmonary tissue as in pneumoconiosis or emphysema will cause pulmonary hypertension.

Disorders of the rate and rhythm of the heart

Figure 3.14 shows the normal conduction pathway of electrical impulses across the heart. In the undiseased heart impulses travel from the sinus node across the heart towards the atrioventricular (AV) node. The AV node splits into two bundles that activate the ventricles.

The sinus node is the main centre for pacing and controlling the heart rate. The AV node and other parts of the heart can also control the rate of the heart, but these are normally overridden by the sinus node. Hence the normal rate and rhythm of the heart is called sinus rate and rhythm.

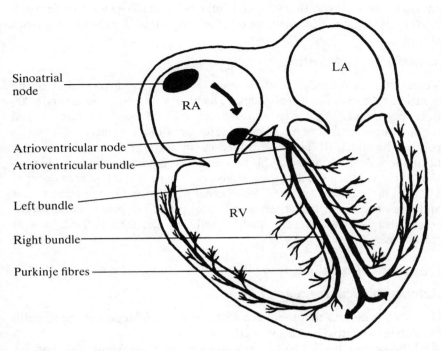

Figure 3.14   Conduction pathway of the heart

Disorders of the sinus rate and rhythm

Sinus tachycardia

In adults, a resting sinus rhythm greater than 100 per minute is described as sinus tachycardia. This rate may be considered 'normal' when the patient is undergoing exercise.

Sinus bradycardia

Sinus bradycardia is a rhythm which is slower than normal. This is taken to be lower than 60 per minute. It occurs abnormally in conditions such as myxoedema or raised intracranial pressure, but in many fit patients this may be considered 'normal'.

Atrial fibrillation(AF)

Irregular atrial impulses may occur at over 250 per minute in episodes of atrial fibrillation. These episodes are related to myocardial infarction and rheumatic heart fever. In myocardial infarcts the episodes are transient and of varying lengths. In rheumatic fever, the atrial fibrillation becomes chronic.

Ventricular tachycardia

Ventricular tachycardia may develop as the pacemaker cells in the ventricle take over the job of pacing. The heart rate may increase up to 200 beats per minute. This may be associated with myocardial infarction and requires urgent treatment. Lignocaine or beta blockers may be given to control the attack. If left uncontrolled the attack may result in ventricular fibrillation. With ventricular fibrillation there is unco-ordinated contraction of the ventricles. The contractions are very irregular and may occur at a rate of up to 300 per minute. Ventricular fibrillation rarely corrects itself and gives rise to cardiac arrest with loss of pulses, respiration and loss of consciousness. The arrest is stopped only by electrical defibrillation or cardiac massage.

Disorders of conduction

Arterioventricular (heart) block

Heart block implies that there is a defect in the conduction of the impulse from atria to ventricles. This is divided into:
(1) First-degree heart block. All impulses reach the ventricles, but are delayed.
(2) Second-degree heart block. Some impulses reach the ventricles, but not all.
(3) Complete heart block. No impulses reach the ventricles.

The Adams-Stokes attack

In an Adams-Stokes attack the patient loses consciousness for short periods of time due to transient loss of blood flow to the brain. This attack may be due to ventricular fibrillation or tachycardia and is associated with second-degree or total heart block. Adams-Stokes attacks can be prevented by the insertion of a permanent pacemaker.

Wolff-Parkinson-White syndrome

Here an alternative path to the AV node is established. This anomalous conduction path allows early contraction of one isolated portion of the ventricle. The remaining ventricle contracts normally. This is usually treated through drugs and/or ablative therapy carried out under fluoroscopic control.

Tumours of the heart

Tumours of the heart are uncommon.

Tumours of the pericardium

These are divided into two types:

(1) Primary tumours. These include fibromas, lipomas and mesotheliomas. Primary tumours of the pericardium are rare.
(2) Secondary tumours. Blood or lymphatic-borne secondaries occur in the pericardium, e.g. melanoma, malignant lymphomas.

Tumours may directly infiltrate from surrounding organs.

Tumours of the endocardium

Benign

(1) Myxoma. This is the commonest primary tumour of the heart. It arises from the endocardium and causes obstruction to blood flow and valve closure.
(2) Rhabdomyoma. This is found in the endocardium as a malformation of the myocardial fibres.

Malignant

(1) Primary. Primary malignant tumours of the endocardium are rare. Rhabdomyosarcomas may exist.
(2) Secondary. Also rare, but may occur as secondary deposits from melanoma or malignant lymphoma.

Diseases of the blood vessels

Arterial disease

As described on p.58, the build-up of atheroma in atherosclerosis causes occlusion of the coronary arteries. Similar processes are found in other arteries. Generalized arteriosclerosis is a common cause of vascular disease. It is estimated that atherosclerosis is found to some degree in most adults over the age of forty. The aorta, coronary arteries, cerebral arteries and the arteries of the lower limbs are the most commonly affected.

Arterial disease in the lower limb

This is one of the commonest areas investigated by angiography in radiography departments. Stenosis and blockage of the lower limb is very common.

Figure 3.15 shows the site where arterial disease most commonly occurs in the lower limbs.

Patients with stenosis of the lower limb arteries experience pain on walking and a decrease in their ability to walk long distances. The pain is due to ischaemia in the areas of the muscles supplied by the affected artery. As the ischaemia and atherosclerosis progress, the patient may begin to limp when walking. These attacks are called intermittent claudication. The diseased blood vessels do not allow adequate perfusion of the muscle during or after exercise. Intermittent claudication is usually associated with the loss of a pulse in the leg. Occlusion of the lower abdominal aorta and thoracic arteries may lead to back pain, confusing diagnosis.

The extent of the damage to the arteries is assessed by femoral angiography and/or doppler studies.

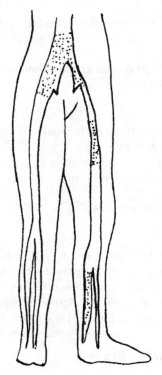

Figure 3.15   Sites where arterial disease most commonly occurs in the lower limbs (shaded)

Gangrene is a complication of atheroma of the leg. This usually occurs at the distal portion of the limbs and may be due to the gradual occlusion of the arteries. Gangrene may also result from infections.

Arterial thrombosis and embolism

A thrombus consists of white and red blood cells and forms where there is a disruption or irregularity of the vessel wall. The thrombus may form due to the presence of atheroma. Fragments of the thrombus may dislodge and form a fragment or embolus. This is carried in the bloodstream until its dimensions prevent further passage, usually at the junction of two or more vessels. This produces a similar effect as found with a block from atheroma. The vessel may require surgery or the embolus may be dissolved under radiographic control.

Veins

Varicose

Veins are described as varicose when they have become dilated and tortuous. Varicose veins are subdivided into:

(1) Primary varicose veins that occur spontaneously.
(2) Secondary varicose veins that occur are due to distal obstruction to venous drainage. Pelvic tumours can obstruct deep venous flow and produce secondary varicose veins.

Varicose veins are also classed by the site at which they occur:

(1) Systemic, usually occuring in the leg veins.
(2) Portal, occurring in the oesophagus, umbilicus or as haemorrhoids.

Varicose veins can be more common in the superficial veins and are commonest in the legs. They are related to obesity, posture, pregnancy and familial factors, and are further complicated by:

(1) Thrombus formation.
(2) Infection (thrombophlebitis).
(3) Embolism.
(4) Haemorrhage.

Thrombophlebitis

This is the formation of thrombus by infection. It most commonly occurs in the legs (95 per cent) and appears as superficial dilated vessels due to widespread emboli. Thrombophlebitis may be seen associated with varicose veins, heart disease, pregnancy or following trauma.

Deep vein thrombosis (DVT)

Formation of a DVT may be fatal in its effect. DVT may occur as a complication of the post-operative period. The site, extent and position of the DVT may be assessed by venography. The limbs are usually affected.

Oedema

The thrombus may produce emboli that lodge in the pulmonary vessels. If pulmonary embolism occurs then this must be quickly and accurately diagnosed by arteriography, isotope scans and changes in ECG.

4
DISEASES OF THE BLOOD

STRUCTURE OF BLOOD

Blood is a connective tissue responsible for carrying oxygen, waste products of metabolism, hormones, antibodies, etc. throughout the body. Blood is composed of plasma (55 per cent) and blood cells (45 per cent). The plasma is mainly composed of water (90 per cent), but also contains:

> Proteins – albumin.
> Foodstuffs – amino acids, glucose.
> Inorganic salts – potassium, calcium, iron, sodium chloride, sodium bicarbonate, etc.
> Waste products – urea, creatinine.
> Blood-clotting factors.
> Enzymes.
> Hormones.

Cell content

There are three basic cell types found in the blood:

(1) Erythrocytes (red blood cells).
(2) Leucocytes (white blood cells).
(3) Thrombocytes (platelets).

Erythrocytes (red blood cells)

These are bi-concave-shaped non-nucleated structures. The red cell count in healthy adults is:

Males 4.4–6.1 × 10^{12}/l.
Females 4.2–5.4 × 10^{12}/l.

Red blood cells are produced in the red bone marrow. In adults this is confined to cancellous bone which is found in the sternum, ribs, vertebrae and skull. Development of red blood cells is called erythropoiesis and is controlled by the hormone erythropoietin which is synthesized by the kidneys and other parts of the body.

The erythrocyte is the mature red cell that forms from a primitive cell called the stem cell (Figure 4.1). Development of the erythrocyte depends upon the presence of a number of chemicals including vitamin B12. As the red cell matures haemoglobin develops in the cytoplasm of the cell. Haemoglobin combines with free oxygen to form oxyhaemoglobin. Haemoglobin levels in the healthy adult are:

Males 13.0–18.0 g/dl.
Females 11.5–16.5 g/dl.

Iron forms the central part of the haemoglobin molecule.

Red blood cells are broken down by the reticulo-endothelial system after about 120 days. This process called haemolysis takes place in many places including the spleen and liver. Iron is extracted from the spent reticulocyte and the remainder of the cell is converted to the pigments biliverdin and bilirubin. These products are excreted by the liver as bile.

Leucocytes (white blood cells)

Leucocytes are nucleated blood cells and are subdivided into two main varieties:

(1) Granular or polymorphonuclear leucocytes.
(2) Non-granular or mononuclear granulocytes.

The total white cell count in healthy adults is 4.0–11.0 × 10^9/l.

Granular leucocytes

Three groups of granulocytes are found in the blood:

(1) Neutrophils. These account for the majority of granular leucocytes (approximately 65 per cent). The level in the adult bloodstream is 2.5–7.5 × 10^9/l.
(2) Basophils.
(3) Eosinophils.

The granular leucocytes are responsible for eliminating micro-organisms by phagocytosis.

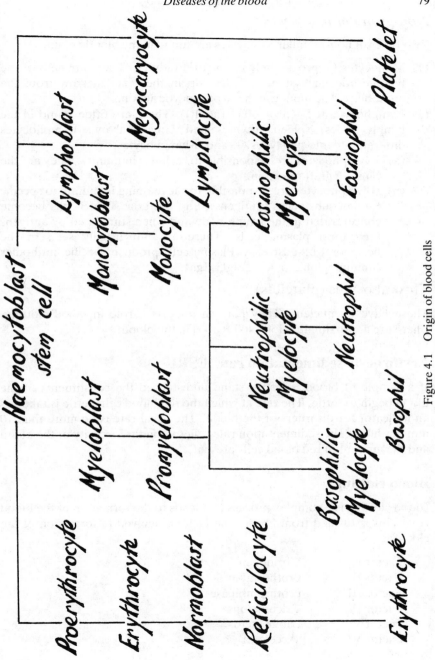

Figure 4.1　Origin of blood cells

Non-granular leucocytes

Two types of non-granular leucocytes are found in the bloodstream:

(1) Monocytes (approximately $0.1 \times 10^9/l$ (adult)). These are cells of the lymphoreticular system and develop in the bone marrow from the monoblast. The monocyte has a phagocytic action.
(2) Lymphocyte ($1.5–4.0 \times 10^9/l$ (adult)). These are often found in the lymph nodes, spleen, thymus and bone marrow. Lymphocytes differentiate into two types, T- and B-lymphocytes:
   (a) T-lymphocytes are responsible for cellular immunity. They are the cause of graft rejection.
   (b) B-lymphocytes are responsible for developing immunity to specific foreign substances (antigens), e.g. bacteria. The B-cells become concentrated in the lymph node and when stimulated by antigens they form plasma cells. These are not usually seen in the peripheral bloodstream. Plasma cells produce specific antibodies (immunoglobulins), e.g. IgG, IgM.

Thrombocytes (platelets)

These have no nucleus. They play an important role in blood clotting. There are approximately $150–400 \times 10^9/l$ in the blood.

Erythrocyte sedimentation rate (ESR)

If a sample of blood is left to stand undisturbed the constituents of the blood begin to settle. The rate at which the red blood cells settle is taken as an indicator for disorders of the blood. The usual rate is no more than 10 mm per hour. The sedimentation rate relies upon the viscosity of the blood and the amount of red blood cells present.

Blood clotting

Blood clotting is a complex process that leads to the formation of the blood clot. This is formed from fibrin. The factors involved in formation of the clot are:

Factor I	Fibrinogen
Factor II	Prothrombin
Factor III	Prothrombinase
Factor IV	Calcium ions
Factor V	Labile factor
Factor VI	'Accelerin'

Factor VII	Stable factor
Factor VIII	Antihaemophilic globulin
Factor IX	Christmas factor
Factor X	Stuart-Prower factor
Factor XI	Plasma thromboplastin antecedent
Factor XII	Hagemen factor
Factor XIII	Fibrin stabilizing factor

Factor VI may not exist, it has never been isolated.

POLYCYTHAEMIA

Polycythaemia is an abnormal increase in the number of red cells present in the blood. The condition is subdivided into primary disease, where the condition occurs in isolation, and secondary polycythaemia, which results from another underlying disease.

Primary (polycythaemia vera)

This disorder is a myeloproliferative disease. This describes a group of disorders that affect the bone marrow causing it to over-produce red blood cells. In some cases of polycythaemia the platelet level also increases.

Myeloproliferative disease has a non-specific effect and may affect other cell elements within the marrow. Over-production of granulocytes (chronic granulocytic leukaemia) and platelets (thrombocythaemia) can also occur.

Polycythaemia vera produces a variety of effects. The onset is usually without warning, the patient presenting with a complication of the disease, e.g. haemorrhage. Disturbance to the circulation supplying the central nervous system commonly causes headaches, dizziness and tinnitus. Thrombosis in veins and arteries may also occur together with pruritis and urticaria. Hepatomegaly and splenomegaly may also be noted.

The condition is diagnosed through blood tests. The blood shows an increase in the red cell count and the level of haemoglobin. The erythrocyte sedimentation rate is shortened.

Treatment

Unless treated the condition may progress to myeloblastic anaemia and may prove fatal due to formation of thrombus and haemorrhage. Treatment of the condition is by:

(1) Venesection (phlebotomy). This involves removal of blood from the

patient to lower the packed cell volume. The blood is removed in small amounts (350–500 cc) over a number of days until the red cell volume is reduced to acceptable levels. This does not cure the condition and is generally used in conjunction with other curative techniques.

(2) Radioisotopes. Radioactive phosphorus (P32) is given intravenously following venesection. The isotope is concentrated in the marrow and acts by suppressing the production of blood cells. This technique carries the risk of leukaemia.

(3) Cytotoxic drugs may also be used to suppress cell production in the marrow. This requires accurate monitoring of the blood count.

Prognosis for people with untreated polycythaemia vera is poor.

Secondary

This is an increase in the red cell volume usually associated with disease. There are many conditions responsible for secondary polycythaemia. These include:

(1) Increase in altitude. Inhabitants of the Andes and other mountain ranges who are adapted to living at low oxygen concentrations show a sustained increase in haemoglobin and the red cell volume. This is a benign condition.

(2) Cardiovascular disease. Shunting of blood from the right to the left side of the heart as in congenital heart disease may cause problems in maintaining oxygen saturation. Pulmonary disease may also produce polycythaemia.

(3) Defective oxygen uptake due to congenitally abnormal haemoglobins. A variety of defective haemoglobins exist that cause severe polycythaemia.

(4) Tumours. Tumours of the kidney, uterus, cerebellum and liver have all been shown to produce polycythaemia. This is due to a stimulated over-production of erythropoietin by the presence of the tumour. This is termed an inappropriate secondary polycythaemia because there is no physiological demand for the increase in the level of red blood cells.

ESSENTIAL THROMBOCYTHAEMIA (PRIMARY THROMBOCYTHAEMIA)

This is a myeloproliferative disorder of the bone marrow that causes a prolonged rise in the platelet count.

The commonest symptom of essential thrombocythaemia is excessive bleeding, usually spontaneous. This usually occurs in the gastrointestinal tract and is often associated with peptic ulceration. Haematuria and spontaneous bruising are also common. In most cases the spleen is enlarged and there is thrombosis of superficial and deep veins of the leg.

Blood tests show a greatly elevated platelet count, e.g. 1,000 per mm^3 of blood, usually associated with a rise in the white cell count. The condition is often difficult to distinguish from other myeloproliferative diseases.

The condition may be treated by irradiation using P32 as an intravenous injection or through the use of cytotoxics, e.g. busulphan.

LEUKAEMIAS

Leukaemia is a neoplastic disease that involves the bone marrow cells. A number of types of leukaemia are recognized and these are broadly subdivided into acute and chronic leukaemias. Acute leukaemias are usually of sudden onset. Chronic leukaemias occur more frequently in the elderly whereas acute types are more common in the young. The incidence of leukaemia is approximately 4 per 100,000 of the total population. The cause of leukaemia is not fully understood. A number of factors are known to cause an increased incidence of leukaemia. These include:

(1) Genetic disorders. Down's syndrome (Trisomy 21) is associated with an increased incidence of acute leukaemia.
(2) Ionizing radiation. Exposure to large doses of ionizing radiation or repeated exposures to small doses of radiation cause an increased incidence of leukaemia. Children exposed to ionizing radiation while in utero also show an increased chance of developing leukaemia.
(3) Some virus infections are also thought to be responsible for leukaemia formation.
(4) Prolonged exposure to some chemicals, e.g. benzene, produces an increase in the incidence of acute leukaemias.

Acute

Types

Acute leukaemia is further divided into two main groups, the lymphoblastic (ALL) and myeloblastic (AML) types. This distinction is made on the basis of response to treatment and prognosis of the disease. Further subdivisions of ALL and AML are made by analysis of the types and structures of cells present in the leukaemia, e.g.:

(1) Myeloblastic leukaemias (AML):
    (a) Poorly differentiated cell types.
    (b) Well differentiated cell types.
(2) Lymphoblastic (ALL):
    (a) Small cell lymphoblastic leukaemia.
    (b) Mixed small and large cell lymphoblastic leukaemia.
    (c) Large cell lymphoblastic leukaemia.

Mechanism

Acute leukaemia is a disease in which there is an accumulation of primitive immature cells within the bone marrow. This leads to the disruption of formation of blood cells. Decreased production of erythrocytes, granulocytes and platelets leads to anaemia and an increased incidence of infection and bleeding. Further disruption to the production of blood cells is caused by involvement of the spleen and lymph nodes. Patients may present with a variety of symptoms. These include:

(1) Nausea and headaches.
(2) Bleeding of the gums and gastrointestinal tract.
(3) Enlargement of the spleen, lymph nodes and liver.
(4) Anaemia is commonly present.
(5) Bone pain due to involvement of the marrow and the joints may also be present.

Diagnosis

The condition is usually diagnosed by taking blood and bone marrow samples. The blood shows anaemia, lowered platelet count and a high white cell count composed of immature white 'blast' cells. The bone marrow shows replacement of healthy bone marrow by immature 'blast' cells. The bone shows an increased cellularity and it may be difficult to aspirate bone marrow. Erythropoiesis is much reduced.

Treatment

Initial treatment of the disease is carried out to counteract the effects of the illness. Thus blood is given to control anaemia and local infections are treated by the use of antibiotics. Cytotoxic drugs are then given to cure the disease. Long-term application of these drugs is necessary to give complete remission. In some cases, e.g. where there is involvement of the central nervous system, irradiation of the whole body or spine is carried out. This is followed by bone marrow transplant to replace the damaged marrow. Complete remission from the disease is achieved when all the leukaemic cells are destroyed.

Prognosis

If untreated the disease is usually fatal. The progress of the illness when treated is variable and may be one illness punctuated by periods of remission. Complete remission depends upon the type of leukaemia present.

Chronic

Chronic leukaemias may be divided into the following types:

(1) Chronic myelocytic leukaemia or chronic granulocytic leukaemia (CML).
(2) Chronic myelomonocytic leukaemia (CMML).
(3) Chronic lymphocytic leukaemia (CLL).

Distinction is made between the various types of chronic leukaemia by considering the type and number of specific cells present and by measuring the white cell count.

Chronic leukaemias may be symptomless and appear as incidental findings:

(1) CML usually presents with anaemia and splenomegaly. At later stages the condition is characterized by lymph node enlargement.
(2) CLL presents in a similar way to CML. CLL also produces defects in the autoimmune system. This may result in persistent infections.
(3) CMML produces infections and a marked tendency to bleed.

Some types of chronic leukaemias have been staged to aid in treatment. CLL has been subdivided into five groups (0–IV) to describe the course of the disease in terms of lymph node involvement and changes in the structure of the blood.

Treatment

Treatment for chronic leukaemias is palliative. Complete remission is not yet possible. The disease is simply controlled to promote a higher quality of life.

With symptomless chronic leukaemia no treatment is given. Other types of chronic leukaemias require more active treatment. As with acute leukaemias supportive therapy is given in the form of blood transfusions and antibiotics to aid recovery from the effects of the disease. Cytotoxic drugs may be given to further palliate the disease. Radiotherapy may be combined with the cytotoxics.

Prognosis

This is variable. In the early stages of chronic leukaemia the prognosis is good. CLL is often non-progressive and has a very good prognosis with minimal treatment. CML carries a less good prognosis with a medium survival rate of approximately forty months.

Multiple myeloma (myelomatosis or plasmocytoma).

Multiple myeloma is a disease resulting from the malignant proliferation of plasma cells. The bone marrow become infiltrated with plasma cells which causes widespread destruction of bone and pathological fractures. The disease is usually restricted to active marrow sites. Plasma cells are responsible for the production of immunoglobulins and the disease is therefore accompanied by an over-production of abnormal immunoglobulins. IgG is commonly affected.

Myelomatosis usually occurs between the ages 50–70, although it is usually of slow onset and may take many years before it is detected.

Diagnosis

The mechanism of the disease is not understood but it is thought to be genetically determined.

The majority of patients present with bone pain and anaemia. Persistent infections are also common due to disruption of the autoimmune system. Renal failure may also occur due to the over-excretion of large amounts of proteins.

Blood tests show anaemia and the presence of abnormal blood cells. Bone marrow samples may show the presence of large amounts of plasma cells. Blood samples usually show high levels of abnormal proteins. One particular type is called the Bence Jones protein which is present in both blood and urine. Percipitation of abnormal proteins in the renal tubules causes renal failure.

Diagnosis is usually based upon radiographic demonstration of bone lesions, e.g. bone destruction and diffuse osteoporosis and abnormal levels of blood protein.

Treatment

Treatment of myeloma is often complicated and there is no cure for generalized disease. Treatment, if given, is usually in the form of cytotoxic drugs. Drugs commonly used are melphalan or cyclophosphamide. Localized radiotherapy may be used with cyctotoxic drugs to cure painful localized lesions. Dialysis may be required in cases of renal failure.

Prognosis

Prognosis is poor. For patients who have received treatment, the median survial rate is approximately three years. Death often occurs through complications of myeloma such as renal failure and chronic generalized infections.

ABNORMALITIES OF HAEMOGLOBIN (HAEMOGLOBINOPATHIES)

Haemoglobin (Hb) is made up from four subgroups. Each subgroup is called a haem molecule. Each haem molecule is a complex protein composed of a long polypeptide chain. Contained within each of the haem molecules is an iron group. In adult haemoglobin (HbA) two types of polypeptide chain are found. These are called alpha (α) and beta (β) chains. The alpha chain contains 141 amino acids and the beta chain 146 amino acids. HbA contains two alpha chains and two beta chains closely combined in a helical structure to produce a complex, tightly packed molecule. The order of the amino acids within each chain is genetically determined.

Normal variations of HbA exist. Haemoglobin A2 (HbA2) consists of two alpha chains and two delta chains. Fetal haemoglobin (HbF) has two alpha chains and two gamma chains. Delta and gamma chains have the same mass as beta chains.

Haemoglobin has a high affinity for oxygen and in combination forms oxyhaemoglobin. The normal configuration of haemoglobin with two pairs of different polypeptide chains is necessary for the efficient uptake of oxygen. Abnormal configurations of haemoglobin produces poor oxygen uptake.

ABNORMAL HAEMOGLOBINS

Sickle cell

Sickle cell haemoglobin (HbS) is produced due to a change in the DNA of the gene responsible for production of the beta polypeptide chains found in adult haemoglobin. The DNA molecule normally correctly codes for all the 146 amino acids within the polypeptide chain. In sickle haemoglobin the faulty gene produces one change in the beta chain and substitutes valine for glutamic acid in the sixth position of the beta polypeptide chain. The alpha chain is unaffected.

This single substitution alters the normal function of the haemoglobin molecule. In its deoxygenated state haemoglobin is normally stable. Deoxygenated sickle haemoglobin is very unstable and has a tendency to crystallize out in the red cell. This causes sickle haemoglobin molecules to aggregate together, giving the cells the characteristic sickle shape. The affected haemoglobin molecules are unable to take up oxygen and cause further problems by obstructing blood flow.

The amount of sickle haemoglobin within the erythrocyte gives a guide to the possibility of the red cell sickling. It is estimated that if 50 per cent of the haemoglobin in the red cell is of the sickle type then the patient will probably by symptomless. People who show symptoms of sickle cell disease tend to have up to 90 per cent of their haemoglobin in the sickle form.

Inheritance

Sickle cell haemoglobin is an inherited characteristic. People inherit the diseased genes that produce sickle haemoglobin in two forms. They may obtain an abnormal haemoglobin gene from each parent. In this case a high proportion of the haemoglobin will be abnormal and the recipient will show symptoms of sickle disease. Alternatively the patient may receive only one abnormal haemoglobin gene. In this case the patient acts as a carrier for the disease and may be symptomless. If two carriers produce offspring then the child will inherit the sickle cell condition (Figure 4.2):

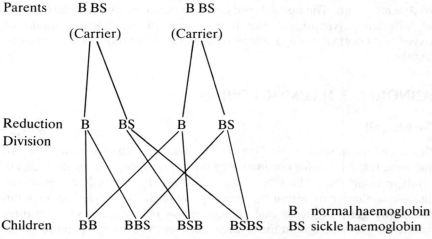

Figure 4.2   Genetic transference of sickle cell haemoglobin

The result of fertilization produces:

50 per cent of the children are carriers (BBS).
25 per cent have normal haemoglobin (BB).
25 per cent have high amounts of sickle haemoglobin (BSBS).

Fetal haemoglobin does not contain beta chains. Adult haemoglobin develops fully within the first few months, therefore sickle disease may not be apparent in the newborn.

Pure sickle cell haemoglobin is predominant in cental Africa.

Sickle cell anaemia

Most patients with sickle cell disease live in comparatively good health. However this is sometimes punctuated by a sickle cell crisis. Many types of crises occur, including the sudden pooling of large quantities of blood in the spleen, a sudden dramatic reduction in the amount of available healthy red blood cells and the suppression of red bone marrow.

Bony changes may be noted in severe cases. Widening of the medullary cavity and loss of trabeculae may be seen. This may be associated with severe bone pain. Enlargement of the spleen may also be found, but this is commoner in children. By adulthood the spleen has become fibrosed due to repeated episodes of infarction caused by the presence of the sickle cells.

The condition is treated by the maintenance of a healthy diet and good general health. If a crisis occurs then treatment may be necessary in the form of oxygen, blood transfusions and analgesia.

Thalassaemia

Thalassaemia describes a group of diseases that are produced by disruption to normal haemoglobin formation. There are two main forms of thalassaemia, alpha and beta. In alpha thalassaemia, production of the alpha polypeptide chain is suppressed, while in beta thalassaemia, the beta chain is absent. Beta thalassaemia is characterized by the continued production of fetal haemoglobin with the substitution of gamma chains for beta chains.

The severity of the conditions is variable and ranges from a complete absence of one type of chain (thalassaemia major) to only a partial absence (thalassaemia minor). The condition is a genetically determined disease and is inherited in a similar way to sickle cell disease.

Carriers of alpha and beta thalassaemia are usually symptomless or possess mild forms of anaemia. Children who inherit beta thalassaemia major develop a variety of conditions. Severe anaemia is common due to depletion in iron levels in the blood. This develops after the child is a few months old, by which time fetal haemoglobin has developed into the adult form. Severe bone changes may also be seen, producing widening of the medullary cavity and pathological fractures.

Some forms of thalassaemia are incompatible with life, e.g. alpha thalassaemia major. The baby dies in utero due to the presence of a haemoglobin molecule with no alpha polypeptide chains present. Fetal haemoglobin has two alpha chains and two gamma chains which in mature blood change to beta chains. Alpha thalassaemia major produces a molecule with four gamma chains. This form, called haemoglobin Bart's, is unable to function as viable haemoglobin and results in fetal death.

Treatment of children with viable forms of thalassaemia require additions to diet to prevent anaemia. In cases of severe thalassaemia blood transfusions may be required.

CONGENITAL DISORDERS OF BLOOD-CLOTTING FACTORS

Haemophilia A

This is a sex-linked recessive condition (Figure 4.3) that is almost exclusively restricted to men. The defective gene is carried on the X chromosome. Male is determined by the configuration XY and female by XX. Haemophilia A is a recessive character and its action is suppressed by a normal functioning gene. Women are therefore able to carry the haemophilia gene without contracting the condition.

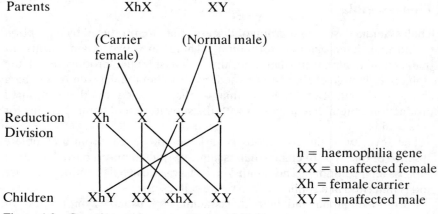

Figure 4.3   Genetic transference of haemophilia A

The chances of a male child being born from the mating of a carrier female and healthy male are 50 per cent.

Haemophilia A is caused by severely reduced amounts of clotting Factor VIII or a complete absence. The condition is subdivided into levels of severity. The most severe cases have less than 1 per cent Factor VIII activity. These cases show the most extensive effects of the disease.

These patients suffer from severe bleeding following mild trauma. This produces extensive haematoma and haemarthrosis (bleeding into the joints). Bleeding into the joints causes pain and stiffness on movement and loss of function. If continued this leads to destruction of the joint. Other effects include peripheral neuropathies and intra-abdominal bleeding.

Diagnosis

Family history indicates whether the male child will be born with haemophilia. Genetic counselling is ofter carried out in families with known, female carriers. Screening of the blood of possible haemophiliacs is also carried out to detect the absence of Factor VIII.

Control

Bleeding episodes are controlled by the administration of large amounts of Factor VIII. Long-term relief is given through repeated doses of Factor VIII (replacement therapy). Large doses of Factor VIII are required and these are available by fractionation of fresh plasma.

Haemophilia B (Christmas disease)

This is a sex-linked recessive disease that is transmitted in a similar way to haemophilia A. The condition is indistinguishable from haemophilia A and presents with all the characteristic signs of bleeding, etc. It is treated with injections of Factor IX. This is also prepared from blood and is a more stable compound than the extract of Factor VIII.

Von Willebrand's disease

This is a condition similar to haemophilia A in that patients with von Willebrand's disease show a lack of Factor VIII. The two differ in the following ways:

(1) Von Willebrand's disease is not a sex-linked condition.
(2) Von Willebrand's disease is a dominant inherited condition and expresses itself in the heterozygote form, i.e. children who inherit one normal Factor VIII gene and one abnormal Factor VIII gene will develop the disease. The disease also has a variable expressivity

occurring with varying degrees of severity. The heterozygote form is less severe than the pure homozygote form.

(3) Von Willebrand's disease is associated with defects in platelet function. This produces an increase in the clotting time.

ANAEMIA

There are many types of anaemia. Some types are outlined below:

Iron deficiency

Iron is essential for healthy living. Seventy per cent of all the iron in the body is held in the haemoglobin where it is combined with oxygen or carbon dioxide in carrying out gaseous exchange. A further 10 per cent is stored in the tissues and is essential for normal tissue respiration. The remaining iron is stored in the liver, spleen and bone marrow as ferritin and haemosiderin. A small quantity is bound to a plasma protein called transferrin that is essential in the control of iron absorption from the bowel.

Approximately 1 mg of iron must be absorbed per day.

Iron deficiency anaemia results from a reduction in the amount of circulating haemoglobin. This may be due to:

(1) Bleeding. In the adult one of the most common causes of iron deficiency is chronic bleeding from the gastrointestinal tract. The commonest sources of gastrointestinal bleeding are hiatus hernia, peptic ulceration, neoplasms and gastritis. Other causes include: varices, polyps, intussusception, volvulus, cholelithiasis, ulcerative colitis and haemorrhoids. Menstrual bleeding and abnormalities of the uterus, e.g. fibroids and neoplasms may also cause iron deficiency anaemia to develop.

(2) Poor diet.

(3) Malabsorption of iron.

(4) Symptoms

The symptoms of iron deficiency anaemia are varied. The condition becomes more apparent as the levels of haemoglobin reduce to low levels. General symptoms include:

(1) Lethargy, fatigue, irritability.

(2) Pallor.

(3) Smooth, shiny, painful tongue (glossitis).

(4) Cracking of the angles of the mouth (cheilitis)

In severe iron deficiency anaemia, the erythrocytes become pale (hypochromic) and small in size (microcytic). The level of haemoglobin is reduced. The amount of plasma iron is also reduced, and this is taken as a measure of the level of transferrin present in the blood and its ability to bind iron.

Treatment

In the case of uncomplicated severe iron deficiency treatment may be in the form of improved diet, oral iron tablets, or, in cases of malabsorption problems, intramuscular injections of iron preparations may be given. If there is an underlying cause for the anaemia, e.g. gastrointestinal bleeding, then surgery may also be required to correct the condition.

Megaloblastic

Megaloblastic anaemia is a term used to cover a variety of anaemias caused by a deficiency in vitamin B12 (cyanocobalamin) or folic acid (pteroylglutamic acid). Folic acid is essential for the synthesis of purines and pyrimidines and the formation of nucleic acids (deoxyribonucleic acid (DNA) and ribonucleic acid (RNA)). Folic acid is therefore essential in cell growth and is found in the red bone marrow where it aids in blood cell formation. Lack of folic acid disrupts blood cell formation.

Lack of vitamin B12 also causes disruption to normal blood cell formation. All types of blood cell may be affected, and affected erythrocytes appear large and irregular and may have structures within them. Bone marrow is also affected and shows the presence of abnormal red cell precursors (megaloblast).

Vitamin B12 is only absorbed in the ileum in combination with intrinsic factor, which is secreted in the gastric juices. Lack of intrinsic factor, a complex molecule with an ability to bind to vitamin B12, leads to no absorption of the vitamin.

Pernicious (Addison's anaemia)

Marked changes to the bowel wall are noted in patients with pernicious anaemia. Biopsy of the stomach wall shows atrophy of the mucosa. This leads to retarded secretion of intrinsic factor and subsequent malabsorption of vitamin B12.

The condition may be caused by:

(1) Antibodies. Biopsy of the stomach wall may show the presence of antibodies to intrinsic factor (auto-antibodies). These block the action of the intrinsic factor.

(2) Pernicious anaemia is genetically determined. The condition tends to occur within family groups.
(3) Surgery to the stomach and ileum may disrupt the uptake of vitamin B12.

Pernicious anaemia is more common in Scandinavian countries and the disease is in general more common in Europeans. This is probably due to a higher incidence of inbreeding. Patients affected by the condition tend to be in the 40–80 year age group with a fair complexion.

The symptoms of pernicious anaemia are those of general megaloblastic anaemias:

(1) Anaemia. The anaemia produces similar effects to that seen in iron deficiency anaemia, e.g. pallor, glossitis, tiredness, etc.
(2) Neurological abnormalities. Degenerative changes occur throughout the nervous system. Inflammation of the nerve fibres and degenerative changes are common. Degeneration of the spinal cord and mental dysfunction may also occur.

Intramuscular injections of vitamin B12 are usually given with good response. The injections must be maintained on a long-term basis and may be given at monthly intervals.

Juvenile pernicious anaemia

This is a megaloblastic anaemia caused by a lack of folic acid.

Secondary

Secondary anaemia is produced as a result of another disease, e.g. renal disease. Chronic renal failure is associated with anaemia. Destruction of kidney tissue associated with renal failure leads to the disruption of the secretion of erythropoietin. The resulting under-stimulation of the bone marrow reduces production of blood cells.

Patients in chronic renal failure also have a tendency to gastrointestinal and gynaecological bleeding. This loss of blood places a heavy demand upon erythropoiesis and contributes significantly to the development of anaemia. Anaemia may also develop in patients who are on renal dialysis. This is also due to disruption of erythropoietin production.

ENDOCRINE DISORDERS

Thyroid disease

There is a connection between hypothyroidism and pernicious anaemia.

This is thought to be an autoimmune process. Antibodies to both intrinsic factor and thyroid hormones are found in the gastric juices of some patients.

Hypopituitarism

Removal of the pituitary gland is known to produce anaemia. This is thought to be due to the absence of secretions from the anterior lobe of the gland, e.g. thyroid-stimulating hormone.

Gonadal dysfunction

Androgens are known to stimulate red cell production. Loss of gonad function may result in anaemia.

Liver disease

Chronic hepatitis may produce increased destruction of erythrocytes.

Bone marrow disease

Depression of bone marrow function following radiotherapy or chemotherapy may produce an aplastic anaemia. Cytotoxic drugs such as procarbazine and vincristine are know to depress marrow function. Secondary malignant disease from the thyroid, melanoma, lung, breast and kidney all produce disruption to bone marrow function and subsequent anaemia. In some cases of severe aplastic anaemia following treatment, e.g. whole body radiotherapy, marrow transplant may be carried out.

PLATELET DEFECTS

Platelets play an important part in the control of bleeding. They seal the site of the injury by releasing clotting factors into the site of bleeding. The healthy adult platelet count is $150-400 \times 10^9/l$. Low platelet counts, e.g. 40 x $10^9/l$ (thrombocytopenia) cause an increased tendency to bleed following minor injuries. Very low levels of platelets may produce spontaneous haemorrhages.

Causes

(1) Chemotherapy. Following chemotherapy the platelet count may be reduced, or abnormal platelets may be produced by the bone marrow. This is as a result of a reduction in the number of megakaryocytes which are the precursors of platelets.

(2) Infections of the bone marrow, e.g. septicaemia. Infections inhibit megakaryocyte maturation.
(3) Metastatic infiltration of the marrow.
(4) Leukaemia.

5
DISEASES OF THE DIGESTIVE SYSTEM

In this chapter on diseases of the alimentary system the following regions are included: the mouth, salivary glands, oesophagus, stomach, intestines and the peritoneum.

THE MOUTH

The boundaries of the mouth (Figure 5.1) are formed: anteriorly by the lips, laterally by the cheeks, inferiorly by the tongue, superiorly by the hard palate and posteriorly by the soft palate. The oral cavity is taken to lie centrally within the gums and teeth. The area lying outside the teeth and gums, but within the lips is described as the vestibule.

The lips are highly vascular structures that surround the orifice of the mouth. They are mainly formed from stratified squamous epithelium.

The cheeks have a similar structure and together with the lips help in the passage of food to the oesophagus, and the formation of speech.

The gums (gingivae) are a continuation of the mucous membrane that lines the mouth. This membrane ensheathes the alveolar margins of the maxillae and mandible and is continuous with the periosteum which lines the sockets of the teeth.

The tongue is a muscular organ covered with a layer of connective tissue. The tongue is composed of intrinsic muscles, which control the shape of the tongue, e.g. during speech, and extrinsic muscles, which control gross movements. It is attached to the floor of the mouth via the frenulum. The tongue is responsible for taste, the manipulation of food and formation of speech.

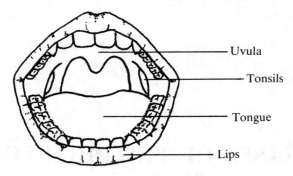

Figure 5.1   The mouth

Hare lip

Failure of the nasal and maxillary processes to fuse causes an abnormality in the upper lip and maxilla. This occurs with varying degrees of severity and may extend into the anterior nares of the nasal cavity.

Cleft palate

Occurs with varying degrees of severity and may be associated with hare lip. In extreme cases both the soft and hard palates are affected. This results in a complete communication between the mouth and nasal cavity. In this case early surgical intervention is required.

THE LIP

Tumours of the lip

Benign tumours rarely occur in the lip. Malignant tumours occur more frequently particulary in the age range of 50–70 years.

Carcinomas of the lower lip are more frequent than the upper lip and are usually of the squamous cell type. The tumour spreads via the lymphatic system, usually to the submandibular and cervical lymph nodes, and by direct invasion of surrounding structures. Approximately 25 per cent of patients develop metastatic nodes.

Treatment for localized primary lesions involves surgical excision of the tumour and external radiotherapy. Spread of the tumour may require a more radical treatment with surgical removal of affected nodes and neck tissue.

Inflammations of the mouth

Oral moniliasis ('thrush')

This disease is caused by the organism *Candida albicans* and is associated with general poor health and with patients undergoing treatment that causes immunosuppression, e.g. cytotoxic drugs. Multiple white patches are seen on the surface of the mucosal lining of the oral cavity. The condition is frequently difficult to control due to the poor state óf health of the patient.

Herpetic stomatitis

This disease is caused by the virus herpes simplex, which exists in a dormant form in many individuals. When activated, usually by other forms of illness, the virus causes fluid-filled vesicles to appear on the lips and mucosa of the mouth and tongue.

Carcinoma of the tongue

When considering carcinoma of the tongue, the tongue is divided into an anterior two-thirds and a posterior one-third.

Anterior two-thirds

Seventy per cent of cancers of the tongue appear in this region. Small localized lesions may be surgically removed or treated by external beam radiotherapy. This gives good results with cure rates of approximately 70 per cent. If the cancer has spread to lymph nodes of the neck then a more radical treatment is carried out involving excision of large areas of neck tissue. Interstitial radiotherapy may also be carried out involving the use of radioactive implants in the tongue.

Posterior one-third

This type of carcinoma to the tongue has a much poorer prognosis, and 50–75 per cent of all cases present with readily palpable cervical nodes, indicating spread of the tumour. Symptoms include dysphagia and speech problems. Treatment involves radiation therapy. Surgical removal of this type of tumour is complex due to the proximity of the larynx. The five-year survival rate for treated cases is approximately 15 per cent. Long-term survival of patients with cancer of the tongue occurs when the lesion is isolated, i.e. restricted to the tongue.

Carcinoma of mouth floor

The average age of occurrence of carcinoma of the floor of the mouth is sixty years. The tumours are usually keratinizing squamous cell carcinomas. They occur more commonly in men. As with most carcinomas localized tumours are more easily treated and respond well to radiation therapy and surgical excision. Spread to the cheeks and other structures involves widespread excision of tissue and reconstructive plastic surgery using skin from the chest wall. Prognosis is poor with a five-year survival rate of approximately 15 per cent.

SALIVARY GLANDS

Three pairs of salivary glands are located outside the mouth (Figure 5.2):

(1) The parotid glands lie to the side of the mandible and empty their secretions into the mouth via Stensen's duct.
(2) The submandibular glands lie beneath the base of the tongue and empty their secretions into the oral cavity via Wharton's duct.
(3) The sublingual glands lie anteriorly to the submandibular gland and empty their secretions into the base of the mouth via a number of ducts.

The salivary glands are mucous-secreting glands.

Imflammations (sialodenitis)

Non-specific inflammations of the salivary glands are thought to arise from direct infection through the duct connecting the gland to the oral cavity. Chronic inflammations produce a scarred lumpy gland that may be diagnosed as calculi or as a tumour. Abscess formation may result from gross infection of the gland. Infection of the gland may also be associated with mumps. This is a viral infection that usually causes swelling of the parotid gland.

Sialolithiasis

Calculi in the ducts of salivary glands most commonly occur in Wharton's duct. The patient becomes aware of pain on eating and the stone is often palpable. Obstruction of the gland causes sialodenitis and impaired function. Long-term obstruction may lead to atrophy of the gland. Sialograms are carried out to demonstrate the position and size of salivary calculi.

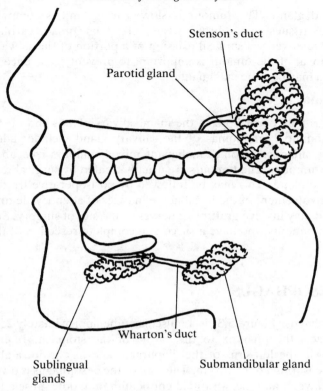

Figure 5.2   Position of the salivary glands

Cysts

Benign cystic lesions occur quite commonly in minor salivary glands. These are small glands that have a salivary function and are found in the oral cavity, pharynx and upper respiratory tract. Cysts occur less frequently in the larger salivary glands, e.g. the submandibular gland.

Tumours

Benign tumours

Benign tumours of the salivary gland are much more frequent than malignant lesions.

Pleiomorphic adenoma

This is also known as a mixed tumour of the salivary gland and it is the most common form of salivary gland tumour, occurring more frequently in the parotid gland. The tumour is slow-growing and is composed of a mixture of tissues, e.g. fibrous tissue, glandular tissue, cartilage. The tumour is removed via surgical excision of a portion of the salivary gland. Total removal of the tumour is important to prevent recurrence. A small proportion may become malignant.

Carcinoma

Carcinomas may occur both in the main salivary glands and in the minor glands. Common carcinomas of the salivary gland include: adenocystic carcinoma, adenocarcinoma, malignant mixed tumours (see above) and acinic cell tumours. The tumours are usually treated by surgical removal of the affected gland. This may be followed by post-operative irradiation of the site. Involvement of the facial nerve in cases of adenocystic tumours of the parotid may involve grafting of nerves to the site of surgery. Survival is greatest in patients who have a successful complete resection of the entire gland.

THE OESOPHAGUS

The oesophagus (Figure 5.3) is a muscular tube approximately 25 cm long and connects the pharynx to the cardia of the stomach. It enters the abdomen via the left crus of the diaphragm and has an intra-abdominal portion measuring about 1.5 cm. The wall of the oesophagus is divided into three cell layers, an inner stratified epithelium, a middle muscle layer and an outer covering epithelium.

Oesophageal atresia and stenosis

Pure congenital atresia or stenosis of the oesophagus is rare. Congenital atresia is more commonly associated with a tracheo-oesophageal fistula. A number of types of oesophageal atresia/tracheo-oesophageal fistula are found in neonates. In the commonest type the oesophagus is divided into upper and lower portions. The upper end of the oesophagus ends in a blind pouch and may fuse with the posterior wall of the trachea, but does not communicate with the trachea. The two portions of the oesophagus are separated by a variable distance and may be joined together by fibrous tissue. The lower portion of the oesophagus fuses with the trachea or with one of the main bronchi, but does not communicate.

The condition is often found associated with other congenital abnormalities including vertebral defects and anal atresia. Therefore, it is thought that the condition of atresia and fistula may be due to a major disruption to

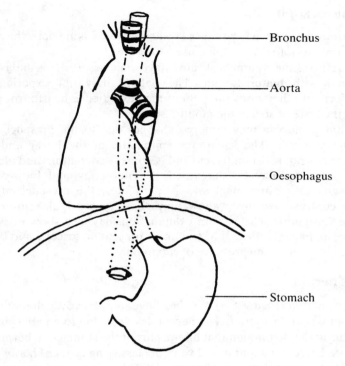

Figure 5.3   Position of the oesophagus

normal tissue growth during development of the fetus. Infants born with this condition require immediate diagnosis and surgery to prevent extensive respiratory damage.

Inflammations

Acute oesophagitis

This condition results from swallowing injurious substances that cause inflammatory changes to the lining of the oesophagus. In extreme cases ulceration and necrosis of the wall may result, with the formation of strictures. Substances that cause oesophagitis include:

(1) Corrosive chemicals, e.g. acids, phenol, alkalis, alcohol.
(2) Upper respiratory tract infections, e.g. streptococcal and viral infections. These infections are not discrete and can invade the oesophagus.
(3) Slow passage of medication due to mechanical obstruction to the movement of solids down the oesophagus.

Chronic oesophagitis

Chronic oesophagitis may be caused by excessive drinking or by the reflux of gastric contents into the oesophagus.

Acid reflux is the commonest cause of chronic oesophagitis and is usually associated with hiatus hernia. The patient may not experience any discomfort. In other cases the patient may experience heartburn, dysphagia and the taste of acid in the mouth.

The lining mucosa may undergo changes due to the presence of acid from the stomach. The squamous epithelium at the lower end of the oesophagus is not resistant to acid and becomes oedematous and ulcerated.

The condition may be diagnosed by endoscopy and biopsy of the oesophagus. A barium meal may help to show the presence of reflux. Double contrast barium swallow may show mucosal ulceration and/or stricture formation. The barium examination may also show evidence of gastro-oesophageal reflux. If a stricture is present endoscopy and biopsy is indicated to exclude the presence of carcinoma.

Hiatus hernia

An hiatus hernia (Figure 5.4) may be congenital, however the majority of hiatus hernias are acquired. The hernia develops due to an abnormality in the hiatus in the diaphragm that allows part of the stomach to herniate into the chest. There are a number of ways of classifying types of hiatus hernia. Two types of hiatus hernia are described below:

(1) Sliding hernia. This involves movement of an undistorted portion of the stomach into the chest. This is thought to be due to a defect within the muscle of the diaphragm.
(2) Para-oesophageal. In this type of hernia a portion of the stomach herniates alongside the oesophagus. This is also called a rolling hernia.

Both types may occur together. Other types of hernia may result from trauma to the abdomen.

Hiatus hernias tend to occur later in life. Many may be long standing and cause the patient no distress. Certain conditions such as kyphosis and obesity prompt hiatus hernia. The patient may experience heartburn, due to acid reflux, and regurgitation of food. In infants hiatus hernia may cause frequent and effortless vomiting.

The condition is usually diagnosed by carrying out a barium meal. The hernia may be demonstrated together with reflux by placing the patient in the Trendelenburg position or by using compression devices.

The condition may be treated by simply controlling diet and prescribing

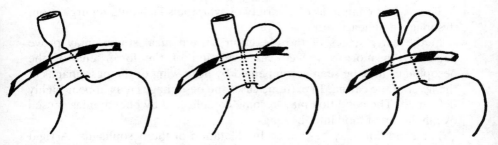

Figure 5.4   Types of hiatus hernia: sliding hiatus hernia (left) and para-
oesophageal/sliding hernia (middle and right)

drugs that control the effects of acid reflux, e.g. tablets containing
magnesium carbonate. Some cases may require repair to the oesophageal
hiatus.

The condition may be complicated by chronic oesophagitis and scarring
to the lower end of the oesophagus. Severe cases may result in stricture
formation requiring dilatation carried out during endoscopy.

Achalasia of the cardia (cardiospasm)

In this condition (Figure 5.5) there is a delay in the emptying of the
oesophageal contents into the stomach due to failure of relaxation of the
oesophago-gastric sphincter. This is caused by an abnormality of the
neurones that control the sphincter. This causes obstruction to the
movement of food into the stomach and a build-up of food in the lower
oesophagus. Lack of motility in the oesophagus further restricts the
movement of food and this may produce dilatation of the lower end of the
oesophagus. In advanced cases the oesophagus may expand to contain up
to a litre of undigested food.

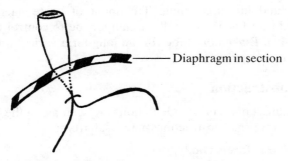

Diaphragm in section

Figure 5.5   Achalasia of the cardia

The patient complains of a variety of symptoms including regurgitation, dysphagia and heartburn.

In the early stages of the condition barium meal studies may prove negative. In more advanced cases dilation of the lower end of the oesophagus may be seen accompanied by narrowing of the oesophagus at the level of the cardia. In extreme cases the oesophagus may appear highly deformed. The condition may become complicated by pneumonias caused by inhalation of food into the lungs.

The condition may be treated by dilatation of the oesophagus. A rigid dilator may be inserted into the oesophagus to stretch open the lower end and thus prevent it causing a severe obstruction. This may only act as a short-term solution and the patient may require repeated dilatations.

Diverticula of the oesophagus

Diverticula of the oesophagus may occur:

(1) As a weakness in the wall of the oesophagus ('pulsion diverticulum').
(2) Lesions lying outside the oesophagus may adhere to the oesophagus and pull at the wall causing a pouch to develop ('traction diverticulum').

Varices

The venous system of the oesophagus forms a plexus that drains partly via the portal and partly via the systemic venous circulations. In some liver diseases portal hypertension develops, e.g. cirrhosis. In portal hypertension the extensive plexus of veins surrounding the oesophagus becomes dilated resulting in the formation of oesophageal varices. These are commonest at the lower end of the oesophagus.

The main danger of patients with varices is the risk of bleeding, which may be severe and life-threatening. Treatment of acute haemorrhage consists of blood transfusion and balloon tamponade to control bleeding, e.g. the Sengstaken-Blakemore tube. In the long-term varices are treated by injection at endoscopy.

Oesophageal obstruction

In the healthy adult a number of indentations are seen along the length of the oesophagus. Abnormal obstructions may result from:

(1) Intraluminal, e.g. foreign body.
(2) Intrinsic (wall of oesophagus), e.g. cancer of the oesophagus.

(3) Extrinsic, e.g. lymph node enlargement due to infiltration of the oesophagus with metastases.

Carcinoma

Carcinoma of the oesophagus accounts for 2 per cent of all malignant disease. The incidence is much higher in Japan, China and Saudia Arabia. The carcinoma is more common in men. It is thought that smoking and alcohol may be causative factors for cancer of the oesophagus.

Squamous cell carcinoma is the most common type of cancer found in the oesophagus. Adenocarcinoma may be seen in the lower end of the oesophagus due to extension of cancer from the stomach.

Oesophagus cancers spread by direct invasion of surrounding structures, e.g. bronchi and mediastinum, and spread throughout the length of the oesophagus. Metastatic spread is initially by the lymphatic system. Later spread is via the bloodstream to the lungs, bones and liver. Approximately half the patients who present with carcinoma of the oesophagus already have secondary spread to the lymphatic system.

The patient usually presents with dysphagia, pain, weight loss and anaemia. In advanced cases the patient may develop pneumonias due to invasion of the bronchi.

Treatment is usually through resection of the tumour when possible. This may be combined with radiotherapy. Better results are achieved for lesions involving the lower end of the oesophagus. Prognosis is poor, on average the five-year survival rate is approximately 5 per cent.

THE STOMACH

The stomach (Figure 5.6) can be subdivided into four sections:

(1) The cardia is a small area of stomach which lies immediately after the oesophago-gastric junction.
(2) The fundus lies beyond the cardia and is taken as that part of the stomach that lies above a line drawn horizontally through the oesophago-gastric junction.
(3) The body comprises approximately two-thirds of the remainder.
(4) The pyloric antrum forms the proximal third of the stomach.

The stomach secretes pepsinogen which is activated in the normal acid medium of the stomach to produce pepsin. Mucus is secreted to protect the stomach.

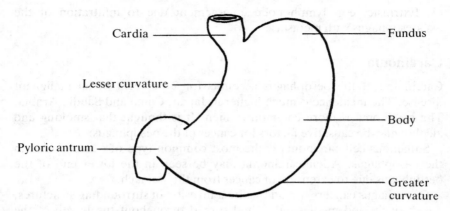

Figure 5.6   The stomach

Congenital conditions

Pyloric stenosis

This condition arises due to severe narrowing of the pyloric sphincter. A bulbous thickening develops around the sphincter due to hypertrophy of the muscles within the sphincter. The thickening extends to the first part of the duodenum. The condition develops at about 4–6 weeks and is commoner in males. The baby develops bouts of projectile vomiting due to severe obstruction at the pyloric sphincter. Surgery is carried out to separate the muscle fibres in the sphincter and allow passage of food into the duodenum.

Anomalies of position

The stomach may lie on the right side of the midline together with the oesophageal diaphragmatic hiatus. This causes no disruption to function.

Peptic ulceration

The term peptic ulcer includes any ulcer that develops in an area directly in contact with gastric juices (composed mainly of pepsin and hydrochloric acid). Therefore peptic ulcers may occur in the oesophagus, stomach and duodenum. Overall duodenal ulcers are more common.

Causes

The cause of peptic ulceration is still not fully understood. Certain factors are thought to promote ulcer formation. These include:

(1) Diet. Lack of roughage in diet combined with 'fast food' is blamed for the incidence of ulceration.
(2) Drugs. Irritative chemicals such as aspirin are known to cause ulcers. Patients undergoing steroid therapy show an increased incidence of peptic ulcers.
(3) Genetic factors are thought to be important in the formation of peptic ulcers.
(4) Gastric juices must be present.
(5) Stress. Stimulation of the vagal nerve increases the secretion of acid in the stomach. It is thought that under stress the vagus is prompted to increase secretion of acid. Thus stress is thought to be connected to ulcer formation.
(6) Smoking.
(7) Alcohol.

Site

Peptic ulcers most commonly occur in the first part of the duodenum and in the lesser curvature of the stomach. Ulcers occur less frequently in the oesophagus following oesophagitis.

Symptoms

The patient usually complains of pain in the epigastric region. The pain typically occurs 2–3 hours after eating when the stomach has emptied and is relieved by eating or drinking. This is particularly noticeable in patients with duodenal ulcers. Vomiting is also associated with peptic ulceration. Small amounts of bile-stained vomit may be produced. This often helps to relieve the gnawing pains associated with peptic ulcers.

Position of the pain within the abdomen may help to indicate the type of ulcer present. Left-sided pain may indicate a gastric ulcer whereas a duodenal ulcer may produce central or right-sided pain.

Diagnosis

The ulcer is usually investigated with a barium meal and endoscopy. If detected on a barium, gastric ulcers seen in profile appear as an erosion into the stomach wall. Seen *en face* the ulcer appears as a rounded concentration of barium. Ulcers in the duodenal cap may be seen as deformities and filling defects in the cap.

Treatment

Treatment of ulcers takes two forms: medical and surgical. Very few patients require surgical intervention (approximately 10 per cent of cases). Most patients are placed on drug therapy.

(1) Medical treatment. A variety of drugs are given to control symptoms. Alkalis may be given to reduce the acidity of the gastric juices. These tend to be short-acting. H2 receptor antagonists, e.g. ranitidine may also be given. These act by reducing the output of gastric juice. They are taken for healing of peptic ulcers and also as preventative drugs to maintain healing. Protection is only guaranteed for as long as the drug is taken.

(2) Surgical. Surgery to relieve the symptoms of peptic ulcer takes two main forms:

    (a) The site of the ulcer may be removed. This may involve a partial gastrectomy.

    (b) A selective vagotomy may be performed. This involves cutting branches of the vagus nerve that supply the stomach. This prevents over-production of gastric juices and allows the stomach to heal.

Complications

Perforation

Perforation of the stomach or duodenum is more likely to occur in acute peptic ulcers. These are of rapid onset and cause severe distress and pain to the patient. Erect radiographs of the chest and abdomen may demonstrate free air within the abdominal cavity. The patient usually requires immediate surgery to repair the affected area. The patient is then reviewed and the extent of any peritonitis is assessed. Follow-up surgery may be indicated.

Pyloric stenosis

Scar tissue associated with peptic ulcers causes the wall of the stomach or duodenum to contract. This may occur at the pylorus or in other regions of the stomach. This complication usually requires surgery to relieve the stenosis.

Haemorrhage

The site of the peptic ulcer may be associated with a branch of the arterial supply to the stomach or duodenum. Erosion of the wall of the artery by the ulcer may cause severe haemorrhage, which may be life-threatening, or slow bleeding over several months resulting in haematemesis.

Gastritis

This is a term applied to generalized inflammation of the stomach. The rugae appear thickened and ulceration may be seen throughout the stomach. Gastritis is generally related to the swallowing of corrosive substances. The condition may also be seen in alcoholics and in attempted suicides who have overdosed on toxic substances.

Tumours

Benign

Benign tumours, e.g. lipomas, fibromas are infrequently found in the stomach.

Carcinoma

The incidence of gastric cancer is variable although it is a common tumour. In Japan it accounts for over half of the deaths caused by cancer. It commonly occurs over the age of sixty and is more frequent in males (2:1).

Cause

The causes of gastric cancers are still not fully understood. Dietary influences are suspected – eating smoked foods is thought to be a contributary factor. Familial and hereditary factors are also thought to be important. Peptic ulcers are not thought to act as precursors of cancer. Some benign tumours, e.g. gastric adenomas, are known to become carcinogenic.

Types

The majority of malignant gastric carcinomas (90 per cent) are adenocarcinomas. These are most frequently found in the pyloric area (60 per cent), the lesser curvature and the cardia. They rarely affect the greater curvature of the stomach.

Symptoms

The patient presents with a variety of symptoms. These may simply be feelings of discomfort and 'indigestion'. In advanced stages pyloric stenosis may develop and the patient may vomit food or blood.

Diagnosis

A barium meal is most commonly used to detect cancer of the stomach. Carcinomas usually produce irregular filling defects, and large craters may be seen in the wall of the stomach. The mucosal folds may also appear highly thickend. In advanced cases of diffuse carcinoma involvement (linitis plastica) the stomach appears narrowed and distorted by the loss of normal mucosa. Endoscopy is also carried out to biopsy suspected lesions. Often the lesion may be readily palpated in the abdomen.

Spread

The tumour may spread by direct invasion of surrounding organs, e.g. the liver and pancreas. Spread may also be via the peritoneum. Secondary involvement of the ovary is common (Krukenberg's tumour). Lymphatic spread takes place along the gastric lymph nodes. Mediastinal and cervical lymph nodes (Virchow's node) may also be involved. Spread via the blood-stream to the liver, lungs and bones also takes place.

Treatment

Gastric carinomas are usually treated by some form of gastrectomy. The extent of the gastrectomy depends upon the stage of the disease. Spread of the tumour may require removal of portions of liver, pancreas and spleen. The use of radiotherapy and chemotherapy in addition to surgery do not usually improve survival. Prognosis depends upon the size, site and early detection of the cancer.

Polyps

Single or multiple polyps may be found in the stomach. These appear as outgrowths of the mucosal lining and may be associated with cysts in the gastric glands. Some polyps may become malignant. Malignant polyps may only be differentiated by biopsy during endoscopy.

THE INTESTINES

The small intestine extends from the pyloric valve to the ileocaecal valve (sphincter) of the colon (Figure 5.7). It is approximately 3.5 metres in length and it is subdivided into the duodenum, jejunum and ileum. The three sections may only be differentiated by microscopic appearance. The small intestine carries out secretory, absorptive and digestive functions.

The large intestine is approximately 1.5 metres long and is subdivided into the caecum, colon, rectum and anal canal. The diameter of the large intestine is greater than the small intestine. The colon is chiefly important for the absorption of water.

Congenital disorders

Hirschsprung's disease

This uncommon condition is due to an area of the bowel failing to develop normal ganglions. The area of aganglionic bowel remains peramently

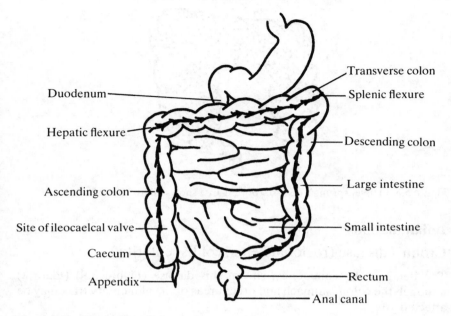

Figure 5.7   The intestines

contracted and causes obstruction of the intestine. This usually affects the upper rectum and causes a widely dilated colon (megacolon) above the point of obstruction (see Figure 5.8). The length of the narrowed portion is variable.

The child may present with acute constipation. The condition may be complicated by perforation of the bowel. A barium enema may be carried out to demonstrate the area of narrowed bowel. However, this is contraindicated if perforation of the bowel is suspected.

Surgery may be carried out to remove the area of affected bowel.

Megacolon

In congenital megacolon the full length of the colon is grossly distended with no apparent cause. The colon becomes overloaded with faeces and the child becomes constipated. Inspection of the rectum helps to differentiate between Hirschsprung's disease and megacolon. In Hirschsprung's disease the rectum is empty, whereas in megacolon the rectum is overloaded with faeces. Congential megacolon is controlled by a prolonged course of treatment for constipation. Barium studies may be carried to demonstrate the calibre of the colon.

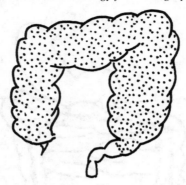

Figure 5.8   Hirschsprung's disease (dotted area shows dilated large bowel)

Inflammations

Crohn's disease (regional ileitis, colitis, enteritis)

The ileum is the commonest site of this disease (Figure 5.9) (Plate 4) although the colon, stomach and other areas of the alimentary tract may be affected.

Cause

No specific cause for Crohn's disease has been found. It is thought that the cause of the disease may be of viral origin.

Appearances

The bowel shows areas of inflammed granulomatous bowel. Areas of affected bowel may be interspersed by areas of normal bowel. These 'skip lesions' characterize Crohn's disease.

Symptoms

The patient may present with abdominal discomfort and repeated episodes of diarrhoea.

Diagnosis

A barium follow-through examination is usually carried out to demonstrate Crohn's disease. The affected areas of bowel show strictures, inflammations of the bowel wall and skip lesions. Some areas of bowel appear very narrow due to oedema of the wall, so that the appearance is known as the 'string sign'. The mucosal pattern may disappear in some areas of the bowel due to gross inflammation of the bowel wall. These areas of gross

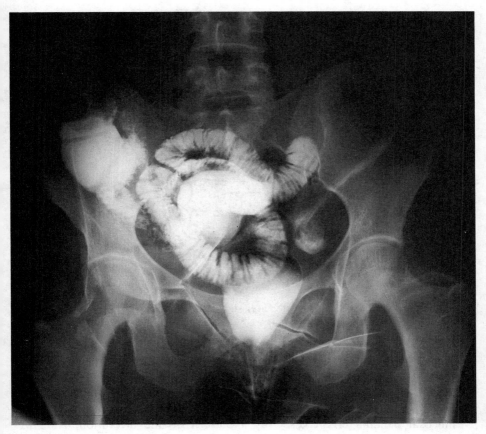

Plate 4   Crohn's disease

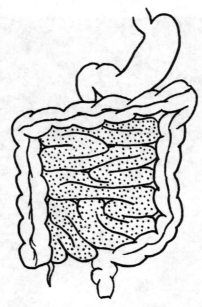

Figure 5.9   Crohn's disease (dotted area shows affected small bowel)

inflammation cause the loops of bowel to separate from each other.

The barium study may also demonstrate fistula formation, e.g. between the bowel and the bladder, and adhesions between the loops of bowel. The bowel wall may develop a cobblestone appearance due to a combination of mucosal oedema criss-crossed by a pattern of fine ulceration. As the disease progresses the ulcers may penetrate deep into the bowel wall and are sometimes described as 'rose thorn' ulcers. Extensive deep ulceration of the bowel wall may give rise to formation of fistulae.

A barium enema may be carried out to exclude Crohn's disease of the large bowel. Colonoscopy and biopsy may also be carried out to confirm diagnosis.

Treatment

Control of the disease is usually by effective control of diet. Patients may be placed on a high protein diet. Surgery may be carried out to relieve obstructions caused by bowel inflammations or to deal with fistulae, adhesions, etc. Some advanced cases may require total colectomy and formation of an ileostomy.

Complications

The disease may be complicated by many factors, including:

(1) Intestinal obstruction.
(2) Formation of fistulae.

Course

The course of the disease is variable. The lesions may heal and not reappear or new sites of infection may occur. Malabsorption is also associated with Crohn's disease and may also cause long-standing problems.

Ulcerative colitis

Ulcerative colitis (Plate 5) is an inflammatory bowel disease of unknown origin and is confined to the colon. It affects all age groups. The disease starts in the rectum and affects variable lengths of the colon (see Figure 5.10). Widespread inflammation and ulceration of the bowel wall is seen.

Symptoms

Symptoms depend upon the site and extent of the disease. In the case of limited bowel involvement the patient may present with constipation which may be easily controlled. In the case of total colitis the patient may suffer from repeated episodes of diarrhoea resulting in dehydration and malnutrition.

Diagnosis

Colonoscopy may be carried out to inspect and biopsy the colon to confirm diagnosis and to differentiate between other inflammatory conditions, e.g. Crohn's disease. A barium enema may also be performed. This characteristically shows loss of the normal pattern of haustra and narrowing and shortening of the colon. In advanced cases the colon has the appearance of a rigid smooth tube. Areas of swollen bowel, known as pseudopolyps, may also be seen projecting into the lumen. Crohn's disease of the colon is usually restricted to the proximal portion of the colon and shows strictures of the bowel wall. Strictures are uncommon in ulcerative colitis.

All invasive techniques are carried out with extreme caution to avoid perforation of the bowel wall. Examination and culture of the stools is also carried out to detect the presence of bacteria.

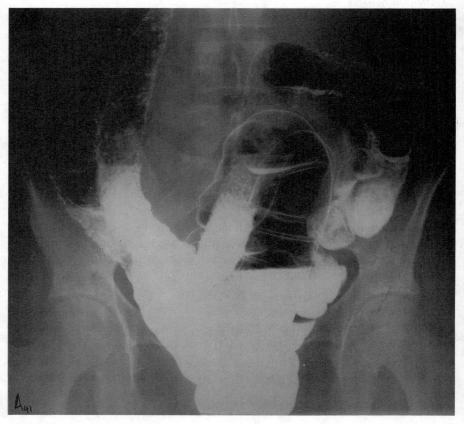

Plate 5   Ulcerative colitis

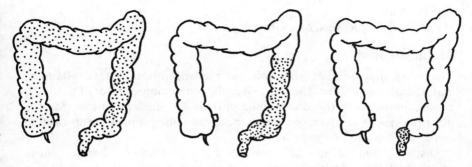

Figure 5.10   Ulcerative colitis (dotted area shows variation in the areas affected by the disease)

Treatment

The condition is usually treated by controlling diarrhoea associated with the condition and by maintaining a normal fluid balance. Steroids may also be given to control inflammation of the bowel. Surgery is required in severe cases for a permanent ileostomy.

Complications

Toxic megacolon. A portion of the colon may become acutely infected and dilated. The wall at this point becomes very thin and is liable to perforation. Radiographs of the abdomen show a hugely dilated and gas-filled colon. This usually requires emergency surgery to remove the affected area of bowel. Barium enema is contraindicated in this acute condition.

Haemorrhage. In ulcerative colitis the bowel wall becomes very fragile and prone to bleeding. In acute phases the stools may show evidence of bleeding. This also leads to the problem of anaemia.

Fistulae and strictures. These do not commonly occur.

Malignancy. There is an increased risk of malignancy in patients with chronic ulcerative colitis.

Malnutrition. Weight loss and disturbances to the electrolyte balance are common complications of ulcerative colitis.

Other causes of inflammations

A number of other conditions cause inflammation of the intestines. These include:

(1) Tuberculosis.
(2) Parasites, e.g. schistosomiasis.

(3) Typhoid.
(4) Bacterial infections, e.g. salmonellae.

Malabsorption

The small intestine is responsible for the absorption of fats, vitamins, water, electrolytes, etc. The extensive villi and numerous folds of the small bowel, particularly the duodenum, provide an efficient surface for the absorption of food. Damage to this surface can cause problems in absorption or the 'malabsorption syndrome'.

Diseases that affect the bowel wall, e.g. Crohn's disease, cause malabsorption, and surgical removal of areas of small bowel due to disease may also prevent absorption.

Some bacteria within the gut are responsible for the synthesis of certain vitamins, e.g. B12. Obstructions within the small bowel may cause loss of the normal bacterial flora within the gut and malabsorption of vitamins.

Coeliac disease

Coeliac disease results from sensitivity to gluten. Gluten is found in the protein portion of wheat and rye flour and in some people causes defective absorption of vitamins, fats, carbohydrates, water and proteins. It is thought that the gluten produces an allergy response in the small bowel, although the precise mechanism is not fully understood. The disease may appear in children as they start to eat bread, or it may appear later in adult life.

Symptoms

The patient may experience chronic diarrhoea and associated weight loss. The stools often appear greasy because they contain a large amount of fat (steatorrhoea). Anaemia is also commonly associated with coeliac disease.

Diagnosis

The symptoms of coeliac disease may mimic a number of other conditions, e.g. pernicious anaemia, ulcerative colitis, malignant disease. Biopsy of the intestine is therefore important for accurate diagnosis. Diagnosis cannot be made on radiological appearances. Barium studies may show the underlying cause of malabsorption, e.g. obstruction, Crohn's disease. General changes in malabsorption seen on barium studies may include: small bowel enlargement, loss of normal bowel patterns and thickened mucosal folds.

Treatment

Treatment is mainly dietary. The patient is placed on a gluten-free diet. Medication may be required to control anaemia and bowel inflammations, particularly in cases of long-standing coeliac disease. Surgery may be indicated in cases of bowel obstruction. Prognosis is excellent.

Diverticular disease

Diverticular disease (Figure 5.11) is caused by a weakness in the colonic musculature. This allows areas of mucosa to herniate through the wall of the bowel. The condition occurs more frequently over the age of fifty years and usually occurs in the sigmoid colon, although the condition may be found throughout the colon.

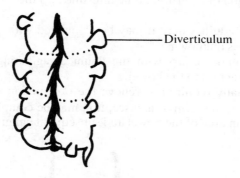

Diverticulum

Figure 5.11   Area of the bowel with diverticula

Symptoms

The condition is usually asymptomatic (diverticulosis). It tends to cause more apparent symptoms when the condition is complicated (diverticulitis), e.g. inflammation of the bowel, perforation of a diverticulum. Perforation may cause haemorrhage and extensive bleeding. The condition may also be complicated by abscess formation, which may lead to the formation of bladder fistulae.

Diagnosis

A double contrast barium enema is usually carried out to demonstrate the condition. The diverticula are seen as barium filled pouches along the bowel. Some areas of bowel may be inflamed and prevent filling of the diverticula. Diverticulosis and diverticulitis cannot be differentiated on radiographic findings, and the condition, when found by radiographic means, is usually referred to as diverticular disease. Perforation of diverticula may be seen as barium outside the colon. Diverticula are often incidental findings on barium enemas carried out on the elderly.

Treatment

In mild cases of diverticular disease a high residue diet may be used to control the condition. If the condition is complicated (approximately 5 per cent) by fistula or stricture formation, surgery is required to repair or resect areas of affected bowel.

Mechanical disorders of the bowel

Intussusception

This is invagination of a portion of the intestine into the lumen of the bowel (Figure 5.12).

This occurs in adults where it may be associated with a tumour, but in infants the cause is unknown.

It most commonly occurs with the ileum invaginating into the colon resulting in obstruction to the bowel.

Surgery is usually required to relieve the obstruction or to remove an associated mass. Long-term intussusception may be complicated by loss of blood supply to an area of the bowel and subsequent gangrene.

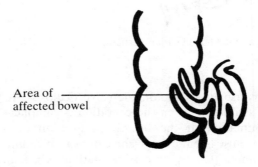

Area of affected bowel

Figure 5.12   Intussusception

Volvulus

A volvulus (Figure 5.13) is a twist in a loop of bowel that causes obstruction to the lumen and the blood supply to the affected region. This occurs most frequently in the small bowel, the sigmoid colon and caecum. It is caused by abnormal adhesions between areas of the bowel and abnormal attachments of mesentry. The patient presents with acute obstruction and usually requires resection of the affected area of the bowel. The condition may be complicated by haemorrhage and gangrene.

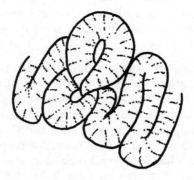

Figure 5.13   Volvulus

Paralytic ileus

This refers to obstruction of the bowel arising from disruption of normal nerve supply to the bowel when no obvious mechanical obstruction is found. This may be caused by:

(1) Hirschsprung's disease, which also affects other areas of the large and small bowel.
(2) Post-operative ileus. This may be short-lived due to disruption caused by surgery. The bowel may recover.
(3) Malignancy. Lesions lying outside the bowel may obliterate the nerve supply to the bowel.

Obstruction

There are numerous causes of obstruction to the movement of the intestinal contents:

(1) Tumours. These may be found in the wall of the bowel lumen or outside the bowel and cause obstruction by reducing the size of the lumen.
(2) Crohn's disease. This may produce grossly inflamed areas of bowel and strictures.
(3) Ulcerative colitis.
(4) Intussusception.
(5) Volvulus.
(6) Paralytic ileus.
(7) Megacolon.
(8) Hernias. The intestine may become obstructed by an external hernia. A portion of bowel may become trapped in the inguinal canal causing

an inguinal hernia. This requires surgery to release the area of trapped bowel. Internal hernias may also cause obstruction, e.g. hiatus hernias.

(9) Adhesions between loops of bowel.

Abdominal obstructions usually require surgery to free the obstructed area of bowel. The patient may be in severe pain or shock. The condition may be complicated by perforation of the bowel and peritonitis.

The stagnant bowel syndrome may develop following obstruction to the small bowel. This may follow stricture formation and causes the normal small bowel flora to bloom and prevent normal absorption of proteins. This is also known as the 'blind loop syndrome' due to its connection with the blind loops of bowel that may develop following surgery for stricture repair.

Tumours of the intestines

Tumours of the small intestine

Carcinoid tumours (carcinoid syndrome)

These are benign tumours of endocrine origin that are found in the small intestine and appendix. They may be associated with other tumours elswhere in the bowel and usually present as intestinal obstructions or as an intussusception.

The tumour is liable to metastasise to the liver and to the regional lymph nodes of the bowel. The tumour has usually spread by the time of diagnosis and produces a number of systemic effects known as the 'carcinoid syndrome'. These include:

(1) Diarrhoea.
(2) Flushing with cyanosis.
(3) Changes to the valves of the heart and thickening of the walls of the chambers of the heart.

Patients with carcinoid tumours have a good prognosis even with metastatic spread. They are most at risk form the effects of the tumour, e.g. systemic changes, intestinal obstruction, etc.

Other benign tumours, e.g. fibromas, may occasionally be found in the small bowel.

Malignant tumours of the small bowel

Malignant tumours of the small bowel are rare and account for approximately 1 per cent of all intestinal carcinomas. Their incidence is distributed evenly throughout the small bowel. It is thought that a number of small bowel carcinomas arise from pre-existing adenomas. The commonest site for carcinomas in the duodenum is the papilla of vater. This may lead to obstructive jaundice. Secondary carcinomas of the small bowel are uncommon.

Tumours of the large intestine

Causes

Polyps. It is thought that specific types of polyps act as precursors to carcinoma of the large bowel.

Many types of polyps are found in the large bowel. Inflammatory 'pseudopolyps' may be seen in conjunction with ulcerative colitis. These are benign, as are metaplastic polyps, which are commonly found in the bowel.

A polyp is thought to have a tendency towards being neoplastic when its structure includes part of the villus component of the bowel wall. Neoplastic polyps account for approximately 50 per cent of all polyps. Their size and distribution is variable. Polyps less than approximately 1 cm are not usually malignant. Multiple polyps are thought to increase the chances of malignancy. In the condition of familial polyposis large numbers of polyps are found throughout the colon and the subsequent risk of malignancy is very high. However, there is no evidence of a correlation between diverticulosis and cancer of the large bowel.

Other factors. Poor diet with lack of sufficient roughage is also thought to increase the incidence of cancers, and certain disease, e.g. ulcerative colitis and familial polypsis (above), are also found to increase the chances of malignancy.

Incidence and distribution

The incidence of large bowel cancers is higher over the age of fifty-five. The distribution of large bowel cancers is:

	%
Rectum	50
Sigmoid colon	20
Right colon	15
Transverse colon	6–8
Descending colon	6–7
Anus	1

(*Source*: UICC, *Manual of Clinical Oncology*, Springer–Verlag, 1982.)

Types

Most cancers of the large bowel are adenocarcinomas. These may have the appearance of a polyp associated with ulceration, but there is however a wide variation in shape and size. Carcinomas of the anal canal are commonly of the squamous cell type.

Effects of the carcinoma

(1) Bleeding. The bowel becomes prone to bleeding in cases of carcinoma and fresh blood may appear in the stools. Anaemia may also become apparent.
(2) Change of bowel habit. Diarrhoea with blood in the stools may indicate a tumour.
(3) Intestinal obstruction. This may develop due to occlusion of the lumen by a tumour. Tumours in the wall of the bowel may cause the haustra to contract and occlude the lumen and obstruct the bowel (purse-string lesion).
(4) Perforation and fistula. Infection of the bowel wall and abscess formation due to the presence of the tumour may cause perforation of the bowel or the formation of fistulae to the bladder and vagina.

Spread

Cancers of the large bowel spread by direct invasion to surrounding organs. Lymphatic spread from the colon tends to be to the peri-aortic nodes. Blood metastases usually spread to the liver. The chest and bones may also be included. This carries a poor prognosis. Spread may also occur throughout the peritoneum. Carcinomas of the anal canal usually spread by lymphatic involvement of the inguinal nodes.

Diagnosis

A palpable mass may be detected in the abdomen. Radiography may be helpful in diagnosing high masses. Sigmoidoscopy is essential for lower masses where barium studies may obscure and confuse smaller masses. Endoscopy is useful in the biopsy and removal of suspected malignant polyps.

Treatment

Surgical removal of the affected area of bowel and involved lymph nodes may be carried out. This may be followed by post-operative radiotherapy. Formation of a colostomy may be necessary. Chemotherapy may be used in some cases.

Cancers of the anal canal require surgery. Cancers of the anus may be treated with a mixture of surgery and radiotherapy.

Prognosis

The five-year survival rate for operable tumours of the large bowel is approximately 40–50 per cent.

THE PERITONEUM

The peritoneal cavity and most of the organs within it are lined and ensheathed by a number of serous membranes known collectively as the peritoneum.

Ascites

Ascites is the condition of free fluid in the peritoneal cavity. This may be as a result of cardiac failure resulting in fluid overload. The condition may cause respiratory distress and may be treated with carefully controlled diuretics.

Peritonitis

This is an inflammation of the peritoneal cavity. Its causes are:

(1) Perforation. Perforation of the bowel due to ulcerative colitis, peptic ulcer, Crohn's disease, etc.
(2) Inflammations. Inflamed bowel and organs, e.g. appendicitis.
(3) Mechanical. Necrosis of areas of bowel due to intussusception, etc. may allow bacteria to pass from the bowel into the peritoneum.

The condition is usually treated by repairing the underlying cause.

Tumours

Primary tumours of all forms are very rare within the peritoneum.

Carcinomatosis peritonei

This condition is due to secondary cancer deposits becoming lodged in the peritoneum. This is often associated with carcinomas of the large bowel, ovary and stomach. The peritoneum fills with exudate which may become bloodstained (malignant ascites).

6
HEPATOBILIARY SYSTEM DISEASES INCLUDING THE PANCREAS

STRUCTURE AND FUNCTION OF THE LIVER AND BILIARY SYSTEM

The liver consists of lobules, all of which have the same structure. A central hepatic vein drains the blood sinusoids. Lying among the sinusoids are the Kupffer cells which are part of the reticuloendothelial system. Lying at the periphery of the lobules are collections of vessels (Figure 6.1). These are composed of bile-collecting ducts, branches of the hepatic artery, portal vein and the lymphatic system.

The functions of the liver include:

(1) Formation of bile. Bile contains bilirubin, which is a product of the breakdown of red blood cells. Retention of bilirubin will produce jaundice.
(2) Manufacture of blood-clotting factors, e.g. Factor VII. Prolongation of the clotting time may indicate liver disease.
(3) Breakdown of protein with the end formation of urea.
(4) Storage of glycogen.

All the waste products of liver metabolism are passed into the bile. The gall bladder (Figure 6.2) concentrates and acts as a store for bile (60–90 cc). It also controls the release of bile into the duodenum. Bile has an important function in emulsifying fats, aiding in their assimilation. Bile is composed from bile pigments, mainly bilirubin, bile acids and cholesterol. These are all waste products. Cholesterol is almost insoluble in water, but is extremely soluble in bile.

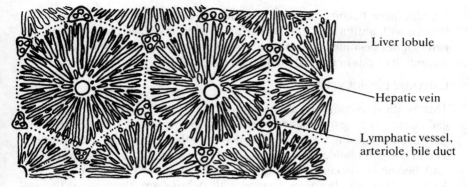

Liver lobule

Hepatic vein

Lymphatic vessel, arteriole, bile duct

Figure 6.1 Structure of a liver lobule

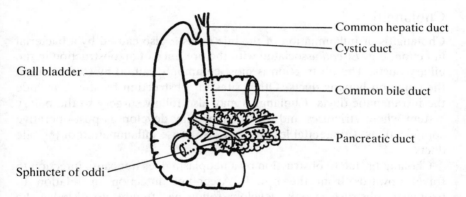

Common hepatic duct

Cystic duct

Gall bladder

Common bile duct

Pancreatic duct

Sphincter of oddi

Figure 6.2 Relationship of the gall bladder and biliary ducts

THE BILIARY SYSTEM

Inflammations

Acute cholecystitis

Cholecystitis or inflammation of the gall bladder is frequently caused by obstruction to the outflow of bile associated with the presence of organisms in the bile, although the mechanism of infection is not fully understood. Calculi in the cystic duct prevent drainage and free movement of the bile.

The patient presents with pain in the right hypochondrium, fever and a raised white cell count. Blood culture reveals the underlying infection.

Many organisms cause cholecystitis, e.g. *E. coli*, streptococci. The gall bladder may become infected via the bloodstream or the bile. Unless treated with antibiotics, e.g. amoxyllin or gentomycin at an early stage, the gall bladder becomes very infected. Without treatment this may lead to the formation of pus in the gall bladder and peritonitis.

Chronic cholecystitis

This is most commonly associated with the long-standing presence of gall-stones. The gall bladder becomes slowly infected due to the stone growing and causing a gradual obstruction to the flow of bile. As with renal calculi the gall bladder becomes scarred by the presence of the stone. The wall becomes thickened and fibrosed and may become cystic and very infected. The bile becomes stained with debris from the wall of the gall bladder. Chronic cholecystitis may follow the acute phase, generally when a stone is not detected in the acute phase of the condition.

Cholangitis

Cholangitis or inflammation of the bile ducts is also caused by a bacterial infection, e.g. *E. coli* associated with the presence of an obstruction in the biliary ducts. The obstruction is most commonly caused by stones within the common hepatic ducts. Other sites for obstruction by stones include the intrahepatic ducts. Cholangitis may also follow surgery to the biliary system where strictures and obstructions may develop as post-operative complications. Congenital lesions may also cause inflammation of the bile ducts.

Cholangitis due to obstruction by a neoplasm does not cause infection to travel upwards from the bowel. Ascending infection in relation to neoplastic obstruction only develops following attempts to dislodge the neoplasm, e.g. endoscopic retrograde choledochopancreatography (ERCP). Cholangitis is therefore a complication of this procedure.

Cholangitis occurs in both acute and chronic phases and must be treated with antibiotic therapy and removal of the obstruction to prevent the spread of infection to other parts of the biliary system.

Gall-stones (Cholelithiasis)

The categories and types of gall-stones (Plate 6) vary and may be subdivided into three groups:

(1) Cholesterol stones. Cholesterol is barely soluble in water, but extremely soluble in bile. Usually the level of cholesterol in the bile is such that it remains dissolved. If the concentration of the cholesterol rises to very high levels the bile becomes supersaturated and the

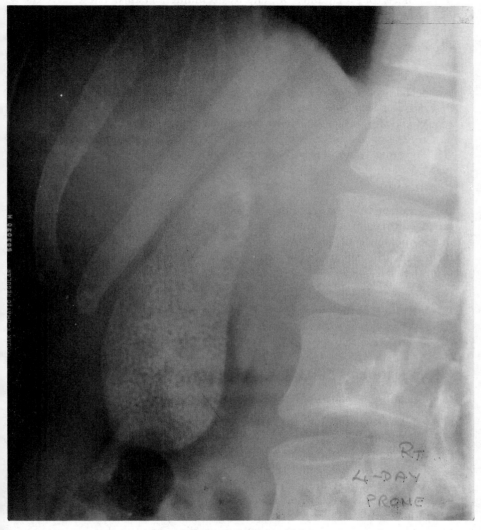

Plate 6   Multiple calculi in the gall bladder

cholesterol precipitates out and forms minute crystals. These have the potential to form stones. Cholesterol stones tend to occur singly and are radiolucent.

(2) Pigment stones. These tend to form when there is an excess of breakdown products passing into the bile. The major constituent of pigment stones tends to be bilirubin. Pigment stones are small and may occur in groups. They may become calcified and are therefore radio-opaque.

(3) Mixed stones. These are the commonest types of stone, composed of a variety of products, e.g. bile pigments, cholesterol and calcium salts. They may occur in groups and are radio-opaque.

Formation

It is a fallacy that the patient most likely to succumb to gall-stones is the fair, fat, forty, fertile, female. This is untrue. However, there is an increase in the incidence of gall-stones with increased age and there is a greater incidence of gall-stones in women. The formation of gall-stones is prompted by:

(1) Supersaturation (as above).
(2) Infections of the biliary system, e.g. *E. coli.*
(3) Over-production of waste products.
(4) Obstruction to the flow of bile.

Complications

Complications depend upon the size and site of the stone, and include:

(1) Cholecystitis due to obstruction of the cystic duct.
(2) Cholangitis.
(3) Obstruction of the common bile duct causing obstructive jaundice. This may produce biliary colic. The patient experiences severe pain if the stone becomes stuck in the common bile duct. The patient vomits and becomes jaundiced. The pain may be referred to the tip of the right scapula away from the right hypochondrium.
(4) Gall-stone ileus. A large gall-stone eroding into the duodenum may cause obstruction of the small bowel. This is an uncommon complication.

Detection

Gall-stones are readily detected by ultrasound or radiography.

Treatment

(1) Medical treatment. This involves giving drugs to reduce the saturation of cholesterol in the bile. Drugs given include chenodeoxycholic acid.
(2) Surgical treatment. Cholecystectomy is often used to remove the gall bladder and prevent further obstruction. Operative choledochogram is carried out to detect stones left in the biliary system.
(3) Endoscopic papillotomy. This is carried out to release stones that are obstructing the lower end of the common bile duct. The common bile duct is cannulated during an ERCP and the opening is cut using diathermy. This allows the stone to pass into the duodenum.

Tumours

Gall bladder

Carcinoma of the gall bladder is uncommon. The tumours are restricted to the elderly and are almost always associated with gall-stones. The tumour spreads to the liver and portal lymph nodes. Secondary spread is to the bones and lungs. Treatment is by cholecystectomy. The prognosis is poor.

Bile ducts

Carcinoma of the bile ducts is rare. When the carcinoma occurs it is commonest in the elderly. The common bile duct is most frequently affected. The patient becomes jaundiced as the common bile duct obstructs. There is a poor prognosis for this type of tumour. Radiology often plays a palliative role in these cases by inserting drainage tubes into the lower end of the common bile duct. These intrahepatic drains help keep the bile duct open and allow the drainage of bile. This relieves jaundice and makes the patient more comfortable.

Jaundice

The normal route of bile formation and excretion is shown in Figure 6.3. Retention of bilirubin in the bloodstream causes jaundice. The skin, ocular sclera and blood vessels become stained yellow due to the affinity of bilirubin to elastic tissue. This gives the illness the common name of yellow jaundice. A number of varieties of jaundice are recognized. Two types of jaundice are outlined below.

Obstructive jaundice

Bilirubin production continues at a normal level but passage of bile from the gall bladder to the intestine is prevented. This leads to retention of bilirubin. Obstruction may be caused by:

(1) Presence of stones in the biliary system.
(2) Tumours of the biliary tract causing obliteration of the lumen of the bile ducts.
(3) Tumours of the head of pancreas that cause obstruction at the lower end of the common bile duct.
(4) Carcinoma of the ampulla of Vater (rare).
(5) Some types of hepatitis.
(6) Some types of cirrhosis.

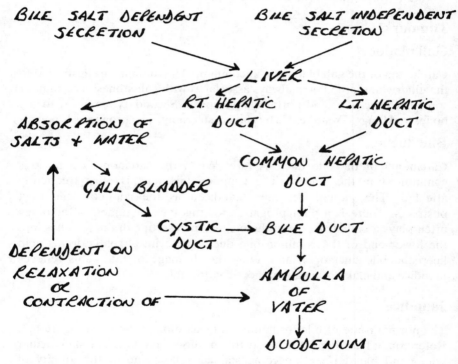

Figure 6.3   Formation and route of bile

Haemolytic jaundice

With this type of jaundice there is an over-production of bilirubin due to the increased breakdown of red blood cells. The liver cells are unable to cope with the increased demand and there is a retention of the bilirubin.

Haemolytic jaundice is associated with diseases that cause an increased breakdown in red blood cells (haemolysis), e.g. haemolytic anaemia. The patient becomes yellow and is prone to formation of pigment gall-stones.

If uncontrolled the retained bilirubin causes severe damage to the liver resulting in cirrhosis, liver failure and vascular disorders.

THE LIVER

Hepatitis

Hepatitis may be caused by viruses, alcohol, drugs and other chemicals.

Viral

Many viruses are capable of causing hepatitis. The viruses most commonly associated with hepatitis are hepatitis A (HAV) and hepatitis B (HBV). A third group, the non-A and non-B types, also cause hepatitis.

Hepatitis A

Hepatitis A virus is spread by poor hygiene. The virus is passed in the stools and is spread by contamination of food, etc. Hepatitis A is responsible for hepatitis epidemics and has occurred after contamination of drinking water with raw sewage.

Hepatitis B (Australian antigen)

This is spread by contact with blood previously infected by hepatitis B virus. It may be spread by blood transfusion or contact with infected needles and syringes. Careful monitoring of blood must be carried out to screen for the virus. This is particularly important in blood transfusion units and renal units. The virus may be passed across mucous membranes and may be spread by sexual intercourse.

Effects

Both types of hepatitis show similar symptoms. Type B tends to be more severe. The severity of the attack is variable. The patient begins to feel unwell and suffers from lack of appetite and general malaise. The patient may then develop a rash and associated itching (urticaria). This initial or prodromal period is followed by the development of jaundice. The symptoms may then ease and appetite return.

Patients with viral hepatitis show marked jaundice due to inflammation and disruption of normal liver cell function (hepatocellular jaundice). Areas of the liver may become necrotic and bile drainage may be interrupted. The patient may also lose their appetite, experience urticaria and suffer from general malaise.

Hepatitis carriers

A large number of healthy people act as carriers of the hepatitis virus. These carriers appear to be immune to the virus they carry. Underdeveloped countries have a particularly high proportion of healthy carriers.

Chronic hepatitis

Chronic hepatitis is usually classified as hepatitis that persists for more than six months. This is a complex condition and may be subdivided into three main types:

(1) Chronic active hepatitis. This has a number of causes including persistent infection with hepatitis B virus, alcohol, drugs and poisons. This type of chronic hepatitis usually progresses to cirrhosis.
(2) Chronic persistent hepatitis. This type has a good prognosis and does not progress to cirrhosis.
(3) Chronic lobular hepatitis. This also has a good prognosis and usually resolves without production of cirrhosis.

Cirrhosis

Cirrhosis of the liver commonly develops following chronic liver disease. Factors responsible for cirrhosis include prolonged infection with hepatitis B virus and long-term alcohol abuse.

The cirrhotic liver is heavily scarred and shows widespread alteration to the normal liver structure. This is due to areas of necrosis that develop within the liver and then heal. This interferes with normal blood flow through the liver and disrupts liver function.

Patients with cirrhosis show abnormal liver function and jaundice.

Liver abscess

Abscess cavities within the liver may develop through blood-borne spread of bacteria from other sites of infection. The patient may become pyrexic and usually complains of pain in the right hypochondrium. The liver may appear enlarged and ultrasound or CT confirms the presence of an abscess cavity. Other causes of liver abscess include the presence of parasites in the liver, e.g. amoeba. The condition is treated with antibiotics together with possible drainage of the abscess cavity.

Tumours

Secondary

Metastatic tumours of the liver are very common and occur in about one-third of all cases of fatal cancers. Secondary tumours spread into the liver most commonly from tumours of the gut, breast and bronchus. The tumour is usually carried via the bloodstream or by direct invasion from surrounding organs, e.g. the gall bladder and bile ducts, pancreas. The extent of the infiltration is variable. The site of the secondaries is usually demonstrated via CT and isotope scanning.

Secondary tumours of the liver complicate the patient's treatment in that the tumours may obstruct venous drainage of the liver and cause portal hypertension with the production of oesophageal varices.

Primary

Benign and malignant primary tumours of the liver (hepatocarcinoma) are uncommon.

Benign

Benign tumours of the liver include haemangiomas. This is a rare tumour of the liver and may occur as a multiple or solitary lesion composed of areas of poorly defined vessels engorged with blood.

Malignant

Malignant primary tumours of the liver are very uncommon in the western races. The tumours are usually associated with:

(1) Infection with hepatitis B virus.
(2) Cirrhosis of the liver.
(3) Alcohol.
(4) Fungi, e.g. *Aspergillus flavus*. This releases a toxin called an aflatoxin which is thought to cause hepatic cancers. *A. flavus* is common in the soil although as a cause of tumours this is rare.

Children suffer from a specific liver tumour called an hepatoblastoma. This is a rare tumour and occurs within the first few years of life. It is highly malignant and has a poor prognosis.

The patient with an hepatic tumour usually presents with jaundice (of the obstructive type), a palpable mass in the right hypochondrium. Presentation is variable.

CT and isotope scans, liver function tests and liver biopsies are carried out to give an accurate diagnosis. Patients with primary liver tumours show high levels of alpha-fetoprotein in their blood serum. This is normally high in the fetal liver, but is low in adults. However, presence of a tumour causes a sudden increase in the level of this substance. Arteriography of the liver is not routinely carried out due to the advent of CT body scanning.

Prognosis of liver cancer is very poor. The tumour is usually treated by resection. Chemotherapy may be used. The tumours are not radio-sensitive.

THE PANCREAS

The pancreas (Figure 6.4) has two main functions:

(1) It secretes enzymes and has a function in aiding digestion of proteins (trypsin, chymotrypsin), lipids (lipase) and carbohydrates (amylase).
(2) It has an endocrine function and secretes insulin (A cells), glucagen (B cells) and somatostatin (D cells).

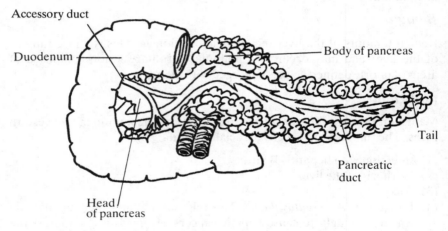

Figure 6.4   The pancreas

Diabetes mellitus

Diabetes mellitus occurs due to a lack or absence of insulin. This results in an increase in the amount of blood glucose (hyperglycaemia). Insulin lowers the level of blood glucose and maintains it at a normal level. Insulin also prevents the formation of glucose from proteins and lipids and promotes the storage of glycogen in the liver and muscles. Diabetes occurs in approximately 2 per cent of the population and can develop at any age.

Diagnosis

Diabetes mellitus may be detected by measuring the blood glucose level and the amount of glucose in the urine. The normal fasting blood glucose level is set at approximately 7 mmol/l. Levels higher than this are usually taken to indicate the presence of disease.

Types

Diabetes is subdivided into two forms:

(1) Insulin dependent. This type is directly associated with destruction of the B cells, which secrete insulin. In the majority of cases the cause of the destruction is unknown. In some cases the destruction is due to chronic inflammations of the pancreas (pancreatitis) which disrupt the pancreas' normal architecture.
(2) Non-insulin dependent. In this type the patient secretes insulin from normal cells but the level secreted is lower than the body requires.

The patient may present with a variety of symptoms:

(1) Weight loss. Lack of insulin prevents the utilization of glucose and the increased breakdown of proteins.
(2) Thirst. This is a result of the loss of large amounts of water. This may be noted in children who suddenly start to drink much more. Dehydration may result unless the level of insulin is corrected.
(3) Polyuria. Lack of insulin produces glucose in the urine (glycosuria). This is associated with an increase in water loss, thus the diabetic patient may present with increased urine production.
(4) Hyperventilation/acetone on breath. Lack of insulin also results in a decrease in the formation of fatty tissue and the increased breakdown of fats (lipolysis). This results in the release of large amounts of fatty acid into the bloodstream. The liver oxidizes these fatty acids to ketone bodies, e.g. acetone and other acidic by-products. These pass into the bloodstream and lower the normal blood pH. To compensate the patient has to hyperventilate to maintain the normal oxygen saturation of the bloodstream. By generating larger amounts of carbon dioxide in hyperventilation, the pH increases. Acetone may be detected on the patient's breath. This is known as diabetic ketoacidosis and is an indication of an acutely low insulin level. This is treated as an emergency as it may lead to unconsciousness and death.

Treatment

The aim of treating diabetes is to control the patient's symptoms and produce the most efficient method of controlling the blood glucose level. This is achieved by one of the following methods:

(1) Diet.
(2) Diet and oral hypoglycaemic drugs.
(3) Diet and insulin.

Diet

Diabetic patients are placed on diets that aim to reduce the level of blood sugar. Non-insulin dependent patients are often overweight and are encouraged to lose weight and restrict their diets. Insulin dependent patients are placed on a controlled, balanced diet. If they overeat the disease becomes difficult to control. If they eat too little the blood sugar level drops beyond a safe level and the patient becomes hypoglycaemic.

Oral hypoglycaemics

This group of drugs is given to patients to reduce the level of blood sugar. They act by either stimulating the production of insulin by the B cells (sulphonylureas, e.g. tolbutamide), or by reducing the output of glucose by the liver (biguanides, e.g. metformin). The sulphonylureas are most commonly available.

Insulin

The dosage and type of insulin given to the patient are individually suited to the patient's needs. Insulin may be derived from animal pancreas, or generated by genetic engineering. Altering the gene sequence in bacteria such as *E. coli* can stimulate the production of human insulin. Patients taking insulin usually inject themselves once or twice a day before mealtimes. The injection may be given into the buttocks, thighs or upper arms.

Hypoglycaemia

Hypoglycaemia is a result of the blood sugar level dropping to very low levels. The patient experiences sweating, hunger and a generalized uneasiness. If the blood sugar remains low the condition may progress with the patient becoming confused and very distressed. The end stage of an hypoglycaemic episode is unconsciousness.

In patients taking insulin, hypoglycaemia usually results from the omission of food or overdose of insulin. The first cause should be considered in relation to radiography departments where patients are frequently asked to stop eating. Therefore diabetic patients should be asked about their diet and injection routines and should be booked at the beginning of imaging lists.

Complications of diabetes

Diabetics frequently suffer from the effects of the disease. The extent of these other effects is dependent upon how well the disease is controlled.

Eyes

After a prolonged history of diabetes most patients will develop a form of retinopathy. Retinopathy describes a number of symptoms including microaneurysms and haemorrhages of the retina. In advanced cases the retina becomes heavily scarred and this may lead to blindness. Diabetic patients may also suffer from increased opacity of the lens (cataracts). This is usually bilateral and progressive. Glaucoma may also develop. This is an increase in the pressure within the eye due to impaired drainage of the aqueous humour. This causes severe disruption to sight.

Kidneys

A large proportion of diabetic patients suffer from damage to their kidneys. Approximately 30 per cent of diabetic patients die from renal failure. Diabetics suffer from a variety of renal nephropathy, e.g. arteriosclerosis. Patients with advanced kidney disease require dialysis and in some cases renal transplant.

Neuropathy

Diabetic patients may develop a diffuse peripheral neuropathy. Loss of sensation commonly occurs in the legs and feet. The patient is unaware of any loss of feeling and may damage the feet and legs without being conscious of the damage. In its most extreme form it may affect the joints, which become disrupted and deformed (Charcot joints).

Blood vessels

The diabetic patient develops atherosclerosis earlier than in non-diabetic patients. Atheroma formation is accelerated in diabetic patients and leads to generalized changes throughout the cardiovascular system. These include the formation of ulcers on the legs and feet, osteomyelitis and, in advanced cases, gangrene.

Pancreatitis

Acute

Acute pancreatitis is a life-threatening condition. It is commonly associated with alcoholism. It is thought that the alcohol stimulates the release of amylase within the pancreas which causes breakdown of the pancreas. The condition may also develop due to the presence of gall-stones. The gall-stones obstruct the drainage of the pancreas and accelerate the symptoms of pancreatitis.

The disease may be complicated by renal failure. In severe cases there is a high rate of mortality.

Pseudocysts are associated with acute pancreatitis. These are fluid-filled spaces that lie outside the substance of the pancreas.

The condition is usually diagnosed by measuring the level of amylase in the blood and urine.

Chronic

Causes of chronic pancreatitis include:

(1) Acute pancreatitis.
(2) Gall-stones.
(3) Alcoholism.

The disease is associated with calcification in the pancreas which may be seen on plain radiographs. The ERCP shows the ducts as dilated and cystic. The patient may develop jaundice due to obstruction of the common bile duct by the inflamed head of the pancreas.

Cysts

Cysts may develop in the pancreas as solitary lesions or in groups, and are diagnosed by ultrasound. The pancreas may be involved in polycystic disease.

Tumours

These occur more commonly in the elderly. Tumours more frequently develop in the head of the pancreas rather than the tail simply because there is more tissue in the head of the pancreas. Three main types of tumour are found in the pancreas:

(1) Islet cell tumours. These are uncommon but are characterized by their ability to secrete a number of substances, e.g. insulin. These are often

benign and produce problems only through their secondary effects, e.g. hypoglycaemia.
(2) Adenocarcinoma. This arises from the duct system of the pancreas. It is the commonest form of pancreatic carcinoma. It often leads to cystic formation (cystadenocarcinoma).
(3) Acinar type. This type of tumour arises from the main parenchyma of the pancreas.

Spread

Both the adenocarcinoma and the acinar type of tumour metastasise:

(1) Via the bloodstream to lungs, bone and liver, etc.
(2) Via the lymphatic system with early spread to remote lymph nodes.
(3) Via direct invasion into surrounding organs and the peritoneum.

Usually, by the time that diagnosis of the tumour has been made, the tumour has already metastasised.

Diagnosis

The position and extent of the cancer are diagnosed by CT and ultrasound scanning. Barium studies of the stomach and duodenum help to show deformities caused by the head of the pancreas. The patient presents with jaundice, severe abdominal pain and back pain. An ERCP may be carried out to show the site of obstruction of the common bile duct. Pancreatitis may present in a similar way to cancer of the pancreas and a biopsy may be carried out to differentiate between the two conditions.

Treatment

Carcinoma of the pancreas has a very poor prognosis. The condition is usually approached with palliative surgery. Removal of part or whole of the pancreas may be carried out together with partial gastrectomy. Surgery to the bile duct is also carried out to alleviate the symptoms of jaundice.
Treatment with chemotherapy and radiotherapy are ineffective in the treatment of this type of cancer. They may be given post-operatively. In some cases intra-operative radiotherapy is given.

7
LYMPHATIC SYSTEM DISEASES INCLUDING THE BREAST

THE LYMPHATIC SYSTEM

Lymphatic tissue is spread throughout the body. Larger accumulations of lymph tissue are found in the spleen and lymph nodes. The lymph nodes (Figure 7.1) vary in size and are connected to the lymph vessels by afferent and efferent vessels. Surrounding the node is a fibrous capsule. Fibrous septae extend from the capsule into the node. The outer cortex of the node consists of tissue that shows high lymphocyte activity. The inner medulla consists of collections of lymphoid cells.

An extensive system of lymph vessels connects the lymph nodes together. The lymph ultimately passes via the thoracic duct into the subclavian vein.

The functions of lymph include:

(1) Production of lymphocytes.
(2) Filtration of lymph with removal of foreign material, e.g. bacteria.
(3) Production of antibodies.

Tumours

Malignant lymphoma

Lymphomas are malignant diseases involving lymphoreticular cells. These are largely confined to the lymph nodes. The lymphomas usually present with enlargement of lymph nodes. However, due to the wide distribution of lymphoreticular cells, lymphomas may develop in many non-lymphatic sites including the lungs, gastrointestinal tract, liver, bone and testes.

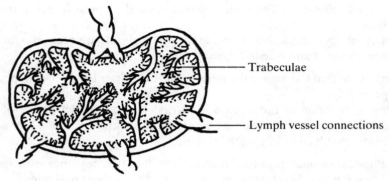

Figure 7.1 A lymph node

Lymphoma describes a large group of malignant tumours that have been subdivided into two groups:

(1) Hodgkin's lymphoma.
(2) Non-Hodgkin's lymphoma.

Subdivision of the types is made on histological findings. Non-Hodgkin's lymphomas are more frequent than the Hodgkin's type.

Hodgkin's disease

The specific cause of Hodgkin's disease is not known. It is thought that the disease is of viral origin. Hodgkin's lymphoma occurs in two specific periods, i.e. between the ages of fifteen and thirty-five years and after the age of fifty-five. The latter group shows the smaller incidence. The condition presents usually as painless enlargement of the lymph nodes. The cervical and supraclavicular nodes are commonly the first areas to be affected.

Diagnosis. Diagnosis is made by biopsy of an affected lymph node. The whole lymph node is usually removed. The diagnosis of the type of Hodgkin's lymphoma present is based on the type of cells present. Lymph nodes with Hodgkin's disease present show Reed-Sternberg cells. These are large cells that replace the normal architecture of the node. There are four types of Hodgkin's lymphoma as based on the Rye classification:

(1) Lymphocyte predominance. In this type the node has a high concentration of lymphocytes within it, together with Reed-Sternberg cells.
(2) Nodular sclerosing. The gland becomes divided by bands of collagen. A variant of the Reed-Sternberg cell is present.

(3) Mixed cellularity. The node is seen to contain typical Reed-Sternberg cells.
(4) Lymphocyte depletion. Here, many atypical cells are present with few lymphocytes and Reed-Sternberg cells.

It is thought that the higher the number of Reed-Sternberg cells the poorer the prognosis.

Staging. Staging of the disease is carried out to find the extent of the condition. This is undertaken by a variety of techniques depending upon the centre involved in staging the disease:

(1) Physical examination for enlarged lymph nodes, together with radiographs of the chest and abdomen are used as the start of staging.
(2) Staging may be carried out by using CT scanning of the chest and abdomen.
(3) Lymphangiography may be combined with CT or used as the sole means to stage the disease.
(4) Laparotomy of the abdomen may also be carried out to show the extent of the disease by biopsy of the liver and spleen. In cases where the disease has spread below the diaphragm, a splenectomy may be performed.
(5) Biopsy of bone is also important in gauging the extent of the disease.

Once the type and extent of the disease have been established, Hodgkin's disease may be subdivided into the following four broad stages:

Stage I. Involvement of a single lymph node region.
Stage II. Involvement of two or more lymph node regions on the same side of the diaphragm.
Stage III. Involvement of lymph node regions on both sides of the diaphragm.
Stage IV. Diffuse involvement of one or more extra-lymphatic organs or tissues with or without lymph node enlargement.

Each category is further subdivided into A and B categories. A indicates that the patient is asymptomatic and B indicates generalized symptoms are present, e.g. weight loss, fever.

Treatment. Hodgkin's disease is treated with radiation therapy, chemotherapy or a combination of the two. Stages I and IIA usually receive radiation therapy or a mix of radiation and chemotherapy. The combination gives a better prognosis. Stages IB, IIB and IIIA may also receive a combination treatment. Stages IIIB and IV are given chemotherapy over an extended period.

Prognosis. Some authorities consider that the histology of the tumour influences the prognosis. Others think that accurate staging of the disease is the most important aspect of the prognosis.

Non-Hodgkin's lymphoma

The cause of this group of lymphomas is not understood, although the incidence of Burkitt's lymphoma has been connected to the Epstein-Barr virus. Non-Hodgkin's lymphoma occurs in the age group 60–70 years and presents with painless lymph node enlargement in a similar way to Hodgkin's disease. However, the disease is usually more advanced than Hodgkin's by the time the patient presents with symptoms. There are usually abnormal lymph nodes on both sides of the diaphragm and spread to extra-lymphatic organs, e.g. the intestine. Hepatomegaly and splenomegaly are also usually present. Fever is often absent.

Diagnosis. Biopsy and classification of non-Hodgkin's lymphoma is not as well documented as Hodgkin's disease. A number of categorizations have been made. The Rappaport classification divides the tumours into:

(1) Well-differentiated lymphocytic.
(2) Poorly differentiated lymphocytic.
(3) Mixed lymphocytic-histiocytic.
(4) Histiocytic.
(5) Undifferentiated.

It is taken that abnormal undifferentiated cells indicate a poor prognosis.

A number of non-Hodgkin's lymphoma are named, including Burkitt's lymphoma. This occurs in children and presents as single or multiple lesions in the jaw.

Treatment. Treatment of non-Hodgkin's lymphoma is more complex than Hodgkin's disease and relies more upon histology, stage of the disease and age of the patient. Patients with localized tumours may be treated with radiotherapy with good results. These types are in the minority. Mixed treatments of chemotherapy and radiotherapy are also used. The prognosis for patients with non-Hodgkin's lymphoma is variable.

Secondary tumours

Secondary tumours of the lymph nodes are very common.

The spleen

The spleen is often involved in both Hodgkin's and non-Hodgkin's lymphomas. Some centres may automatically perform a splenectomy when lymphoma is diagnosed.

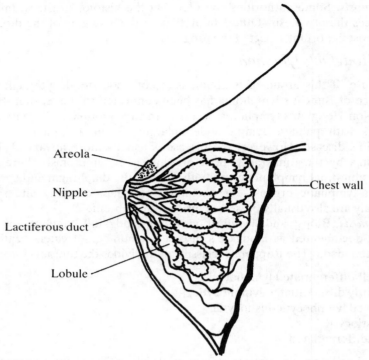

Figure 7.2   Cross-section of the breast

THE BREAST (Figure 7.2)

Mammary dysplasia

This is one of the commonest breast lesions. The condition is affected by the cyclical changes of the ovary. Varying amounts of the hormones oestrogen and progesterone produce changes in the uterus and the breast lobules. These changes subside at the end of each cycle. The condition may be unilateral or bilateral. The patient may experience pain or may be pain free. A number of changes of the breast may be seen:

(1) Ducts within the breast may become enlarged and form cysts.
(2) Fibrosis may occur with the increased formation of fibrous tissue.
(3) Adenosis may also occur with the increase of cell numbers within the breast. This may be accompanied by an increase in the amount of connective tissue within the breast, which leads to distortion of the

normal breast pattern. These changes become exaggerated in the years prior to the menopause when hormonal changes are liable to wide and imbalanced fluctuations. This leaves the breast in an abnormal state producing lumpy, granular or cystic breasts. Patients with mammary dysplasia show an increased risk of breast carcinoma.

Benign tumours

Fibroadenoma

This type of lesion is associated with younger women. There may be single or multiple nodules within the breast. The nodules contain tissues that show hyperplastic (increased growth) changes of normal tissue. The nodules become increasingly dense and sclerotic with age. For this reason they are removed. They do not produce carcinomas.

Papilloma

These occur as single lesions in the main ducts of the breast. The duct becomes distended and causes breast enlargement. There may be a discharge of blood from the nipple. The condition may be accompanied by cystic formation. Most papillomas remain benign.

Carcinoma

Carcinoma of the breast is the commonest form of carcinoma of women in many countries. In Great Britain there are 25–30 deaths per 100,000 per year. The frequency of breast cancer is increasing. This is thought to be due to the increase in the average length of life following on better health care.

The cancer occurs within the age range of 40–70 and is rare under the age of thirty. Breast cancer is very rare in men.

Causes

The causes of carcinoma of the breast are not fully understood. Many factors have been implicated:

(1) Parity. Women who have had children show a lower incidence of breast cancer than women who have had no children (nulliparae). It is thought that the greater the number of pregnancies, the lower the risk. Infertile women are at a greater risk than fertile women.

(2) Heredity. Female relatives of women with breast cancer show an increased risk of breast cancer.

(3) Menstruation. An early menopause is thought to increase the risk of breast cancer.
(4) Precursors. Mammary dysplasia and other cystic changes are thought to increase the risk of breast cancer.

Many other factors have also been implicated, including (1) exposure to radiation, e.g. mammography, radiotherapy and (2) diet.

Pathology

Carcinomas of the breast may arise from any region of the breast. The classification of the tumour type is complex and has many subdivisions. The majority of breast cancers arise from the epithelium of the ducts or lobules of the breast. The carcinomas vary in size from a few millimetres in diameter up to several centimetres in diameter. They are subdivided into the following types:

(1) Not otherwise specified (NOS). This is the most common group of cancers of the breast (60 per cent). This group includes the types of carcinomas described as intraduct or comedocarcinomas and scirrhous. The intraduct type affects numerous ducts. When the surface of the breast is cut material may be expressed from the breast.
(2) Medullary. These are less common than the NOS type (5 per cent) and less aggressive.
(3) Others. A number of other carcinomas are recognized including papillary, gelatinous, mucoid, etc. These account for approximately 2 per cent of all carcinomas of the breast.

Breast carcinomas may be further subdivided by fine histological analysis into non-invasive or *in situ* tumours and invasive tumours.

Spread

A breast carcinoma may take years to grow to a point at which it becomes detectable. Lobular carcinoma *in situ* is a type of non-invasive tumour that characteristically takes long periods to grow to a detectable size.

Carcinomas of the breast spread commonly by the blood and lymphatic system. Local invasion of lymph nodes first takes place. Spread is then to the axillary nodes and on to the supraclavicular nodes. Metastases may then spread to the venous circulation. The spread may also include mediastinal and abdominal lymph nodes. Spread of the tumour via the bloodstream is commonly to the bones, lungs, liver and brain. Direct invasion of muscles and surrounding tissue may also take place resulting in ulceration and adhesion to the chest wall.

Detection

Self-examination has proved invaluable in the detection of early breast carcinomas. Improved techniques in mammography and the use of xerography have also aided in diagnosis. Mass screening using mammography, particularly in America where the incidence of breast cancer is high, has helped to detect early lesions. Once a lump has been detected through examination biopsy of the lesion takes place. Aspiration of fluid usually indicates cystic lesions. Solid lesions may indicate a more serious condition and require removal. Biopsy may be carried out on an outpatient basis or as a surgical technique. Surgery to remove the lump may proceed to removal of the breast if a malignancy is detected.

Staging

Staging of carcinoma of the breast is carried out in a number of ways. One method is outlined below:

Stage I. The tumour is confined to the breast, and there is no fixation to skin or other tissue. Axillary and mammary lymph nodes are not involved.

Stage II. The tumour is within the breast and may have fixed to surrounding tissue. There is extension to axillary or internal mammary lymph nodes.

Stage III. Tumour has extended via metastases.

Treatment

Treatment is dependent upon the extent of the cancer and histology of the tumour. Surgery is usually involved in controlling the cancer. It is estimated that approximately 50 per cent of patients have lymph node involvement at the time of detection. Therefore, surgery to remove the lesion also involves removal of some lymph nodes together with the mass.

Surgery may involve mastectomy or radical mastectomy which includes breast, lymph nodes and muscle. Post-operative radiotherapy and in some cases long-term chemotherapy may be given following mastectomy. Some centres use less extensive surgery, removing the lesion and part of the breast and then using external radiotherapy and needle implants to the remaining breast.

Prognosis

Survival relies upon early detection and the degree of spread of the tumour to lymph nodes. Non-invasive tumours with no axillary lymph node involvement have the best prognosis.

Male breast lesions

These are rare lesions (1 per cent the rate of incidence of females). However fibroadenomas and hyperplasia of the breast may occasionally occur.

8
DISEASES OF THE NERVOUS SYSTEM INCLUDING THE EYE AND EAR

BASIC ANATOMY

The nervous system is divided into the central nervous system (CNS) and the peripheral nervous system. The central nervous system may be subdivided into the brain and spinal cord.

The spinal cord

The spinal cord fills most of the vertebral canal and runs from the level of the cranial border of the atlas to approximately the level of the first or second lumbar vertebrae.

The spinal cord is enclosed within three membranes or meninges. The innermost membrane is called the pia mater. The middle membrane is called the arachnoid mater, and the outer membrane the dura mater. These are separated by the subdural and subarachnoid spaces. The subarachnoid space is filled with cerebrospinal fluid. The membranes are continuous over the surface of the brain. The spinal cord ends caudally at the conus medullaris. Cranially, the spinal cord is continuous with the medulla oblongata.

In cross-section (Figure 8.1) can be seen the grey matter lying at the centre of the cord surrounded by the white matter. The grey matter is mainly formed from neurone cell bodies while the white matter is formed from myelinated nerve fibres. The white matter carries impulses to and from the brain.

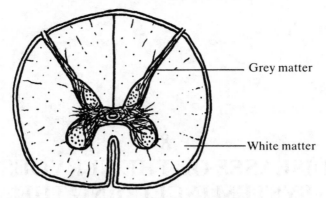

Figure 8.1   Cross-section of the spinal cord

The brain

This is contained within the skull and is subdivided (Figure 8.2) into:

Cerebrum

This is further subdivided into two hemispheres by the longitudinal fissure of the cerebrum and contains the falx cerebri, a fold of dura mater. The two hemispheres are connected by the corpus callosum. The hemispheres are further divided into frontal, parietal, temporal and occipital lobes. The outer part of each hemisphere is covered by grey matter arranged in a number of folds called gyri which are separated by sulci or fissures.

The cerebral cortex is highly developed and contains motor and sensory areas that initiate motor responses and perceive general responses. The cortex is responsible for speech, hearing, sight, etc.

Basal ganglia

These lie deep within the cerebral hemispheres and brain stem. The functions of the basal ganglia are complex and they are the object of much research. The basal ganglia include:

(1) The caudate nucleus. This initiates and regulates gross movements.
(2) The substantia nigra. This is responsible for the control of muscle tension. Damage to this area causes uncontrolled oscillatory movements of the limbs.
(3) Red nucleus. This has some control in maintenance of posture.
(4) The thalamus. This has a sensory function and also has some control over movement.

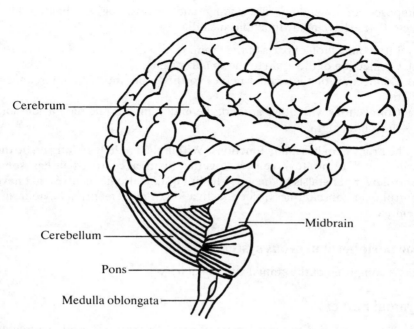

Figure 8.2   The brain

The basal ganglia as a whole play an essential role in the smooth co-ordination of balance.

Cerebellum

The cerebellum lies within the posterior cranial fossa. It is composed of two hemispheres separated by the median vermis. The tentorium cerebelli separates the cerebellum from the cerebral hemispheres. The cerebellum is closely related to the pons and is continuous with the brain stem via the superior, middle and inferior cerebellar peduncles.

As with the cerebrum, the cerebellum has a core of white matter and an outer covering of grey matter, the reverse to that found in the brain stem.

The main function of the cerebellum is in maintaining equilibrium. The cerebellum modulates afferent somatic sensory information and correlates this with the motor output from the cerebrum and brain stem. Thus the cerebellum is responsible for co-ordinating accurate movements.

Brain stem

The brain stem includes the midbrain, pons and medulla oblongata and is composed of ascending, descending and decussating myelinated fibre tracts. These have many functions including:

(1) Interconnection of parts of the brain.
(2) Connection of the brain to the spinal cord.
(3) Connection of the cranial nerves to the brain and their interconnection.
(4) Connections with other areas of the midbrain, e.g. the red nucleus and substantia nigra.

The brain stem has many functions. Within the medulla oblongata lie the cardiac and respiratory centres together with a centre that has some control over peristalsis of the gut. The brain stem also has centres that have control over consciousness, sleep, activation of movement, behaviour and memory.

The peripheral nervous system

This is composed of the cranial and spinal nerves.

Cranial nerves

The brain gives rise to twelve pairs of cranial nerves. These have mainly motor or sensory functions. Spinal nerves contain motor (anterior roots) and sensory (posterior roots) components.

Spinal nerves

The spinal cord gives rise to 31 pairs of spinal nerves. There are 8 cervical, 12 thoracic, 5 lumbar, 5 sacral and 1 coccygeal nerve pairs. Each nerve arises via a ventral and dorsal route which join as the nerves pass through the intervertebral foramina. The nerves give rise to dorsal and ventral rami that communicate with the autonomic system. In the area of the limbs the ventral rami group into plexuses before distributing peripherally. Three major plexuses are formed: the cervical, brachial and lumbosacral.

Circulation of cerebrospinal fluid (CSF)

The subarachnoid space and the ventricles of the brain are filled with CSF. The CSF maintains the central nervous system in a constant controlled environment. It is a completely clear, colourless fluid, similar to plasma and is composed of:

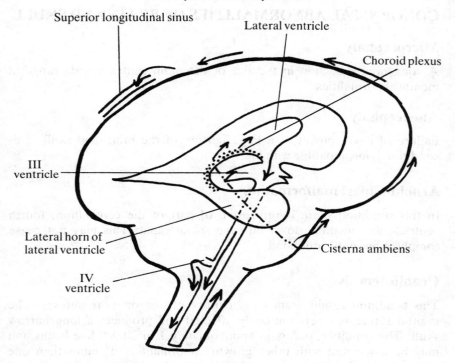

Figure 8.3 Circulation of cerebrospinal fluid

Protein: 0.015–0.45 g/l
Glucose: 2.75–4.4 mmol/l
Cells: less than 5 lymphocytes per mm^3.

(Slight variations in these figures are found between various authorities.)

Figure 8.3 shows the circulation of the CSF. The CSF is secreted by the choroid plexuses situated in the lateral, third and fourth ventricles. The majority is produced in the lateral ventricles and passes via the foramen of Monro into the third ventricle. It then passes into the fourth ventricle via the aqueduct of Sylvius. The CSF escapes into the basal cisterns via the median foramen of Magendie and the lateral foramina of Luschka. Most of the fluid then flows up over the cerebral hemispheres via the cisterna ambiens. CSF also flows into the subarachnoid space surrounding the spinal cord. CSF reabsorption is mainly by the superior, longitudinal and other dural sinuses.

CONGENITAL ABNORMALITIES OF BRAIN AND SKULL

Microcephaly

A congenital reduction in the size of the brain causes a wide range of mental abnormalities.

Anencephaly

Failure of development of a large portion of the brain and skull. This condition is incompatible with life.

Arnold-Chiari malformation

In this condition there is protrusion of part of the cerebellum, fourth ventricle and medulla down into the spinal canal. This may not cause complications until adulthood.

Craniostenosis

This condition results from early closure of one or more sutures. The sagittal suture is most commonly affected and produces a long narrow skull. The condition occurs in approximately 1 in 20,000 live births and may be associated with other growth abnormalities. If more than one suture is involved surgery to the skull is required to prevent raised intracranial pressure. Unless corrected the raised intracranial pressure may cause severe abnormalities, e.g. blindness. The condition may be corrected by the creation of false sutures within the skull vault. Prognosis is good unless the condition is complicated by hydrocephalus or by other growth anomalies.

Hydrocephalus

This is defined as an excessive amount of cerebrospinal fluid. The commonest cause is an obstruction to the flow of CSF. Two types of hydrocephalus are recognized:

(1) Communicating. This implies that although hydrocephalus is present there is still communication between the ventricles and the subarachnoid space. Thus CSF is free to travel down into the spinal canal but cannot travel upwards over the cerebral hemispheres to the arachnoid villi where CSF is reabsorbed. The obstruction is therefore at the base of the brain in the basal cisterns blocking the cisterna albiens.

(2) Non-communicating. This type of hydrocephalus is due to a block within the ventricular system preventing CSF from passing into the subarachnoid space. The block occurs most commonly at the foramen of Monro, the aqueduct of Sylvius or at the drainage point of the fourth ventricle.

Congenital

Both communicating and non-communicating hydrocephalus may be congenital. Congenital hydrocephalus is present at birth or develops soon after. The condition may be caused by:

(1) Intra-uterine infections or trauma to the baby at birth. Infections, e.g. meningitis, may cause adhesions between cell surfaces that lead to mechanical obstructions of the CSF.
(2) Anatomical abnormalities (approximately 25 per cent of all cases), e.g. narrowing of the aqueduct of Sylvius, Arnold-Chiari malformation.
(3) Tumours. Obstruction due to tumours occurs in a few cases.
(4) Over-production of CSF.

Clinical features

The retention of excess CSF causes the brain to expand against the skull. This causes an increase in the size of the head, increase in the width and tension of the fontanelles and increased prominence of the veins on the scalp. The face may also appear dwarfed by the size of the skull vault. The circumference of the child's skull may be checked against a readily available chart. This chart plots the upper and lower limits and the mean head circumference against age. At birth the mean normal head circumference is 35 cm; at six months this is expected to have risen to 43 cm.

Diagnosis

Radiography of the skull may help to demonstrate widened fontanelles, but the condition is usually confirmed by CT scanning. This is an accurate non-invasive technique that demonstrates which ventricles are dilated and the site of the lesion. Obstruction to the foramen of Monro causes the lateral ventricles to dilate. Obstruction of the aqueduct of Sylvius causes involvement of the third ventricle. Obstructions below the level of the fourth ventricle will also cause this ventricle to dilate. Radiography of the skull may help to demonstrate widened fontanelles.

Outcome

Unless diagnosed and treated early the child may suffer from physical and mental abnormalities. It is thought that these disabilities are not simply due to damage to the cerebral cortex caused by expansion of the ventricles, but due to pre-existing brain damage. It is estimated that only 25 per cent of those cases diagnosed within the first three months of life survive into adulthood. In some cases the hydrocephalus undergoes a natural arrest with little or no impairment to mental and physical functions. Disabilities as a result of hydrocephalus include mental retardation, blindness and spasticity.

Treatment

Congenital hydrocephalus is treated by surgery. Various operations are currently performed.

Shunt. A number of shunting operations are carried out to divert CSF away from the brain to other body cavities where it is absorbed:

(1) Ventriculo-peritoneal shunt. This involves placing a drainage tube in the lateral ventricle via a burr hole (an opening through the bone of the skull). The tube is then burrowed subcutaneously down through the neck and chest and placed in the peritoneum above the level of the liver. This is the simplest method of drainage and may be modified with the addition of a valve to control the rate of drainage of CSF.
(2) Ventriculo-caval shunt. This system involves drainage of the CSF from the brain into the vascular system. A drainage tube is inserted into the lateral ventricle and directed down through the internal jugular vein into the superior vena cava. To prevent reflux of blood up into the ventricles, a one-way valve is placed in the system. The valve may be placed behind the ear and opens when pressure within the ventricular system rises above a preset point. The size of valve varies depending upon the age of the child.

Removal of obstruction. Surgical attempts may be made to remove the obstruction to CSF drainage. This is carried out in cases of structural malformations.

Shunting is used for communicating and non-communicating forms of hydrocephalus. The shunt may only need to be used as a short-term measure after which the hydrocephalus resolves due to development of normal drainage pathways.

The drainage tubes are usually radio-opaque and their position may be checked using radiography. Skull, neck films, chest, abdominal radiographs and CT scanning are used to show the course and position of the ends of the tube. CT scanning will also check resolution of hydrocephalus and detect other complications, e.g. subdural haematoma. In some cases the tube may become blocked or infected. Infection of the tubing usually results in removal of all or part of the drainage system.

Acquired

This may be caused by:

(1) Narrowing of the aqueduct of Sylvius lying between the third and fourth ventricles.
(2) Obstruction to the flow of CSF by the presence of tumours, particularly at the level of the third and fourth ventricles.
(3) Late manifestation of anatomical defects.
(4) Head injuries.
(5) Infections.

Unlike children, where the fontanelles are open, the fused sutures of the adult cranium do not permit expansion of the skull to accommodate the rise in intracranial pressure associated with hydrocephalus. In long-standing adult or teenage hydrocephalus this may result in blindness. This is due to raised intracranial pressure in the subarachnoid space surrounding the optic nerves (papilloedema) that compresses the optic nerves and leads eventually to atrophy. Skull radiographs may also show other results of raised intracranial pressure. Erosion of the dorsum sellae and expansion of the pituitary fossa are common.

Adult hydrocephalus is treated by carrying out a bypass operation to redirect the CSF around the area of the block or narrowing. This operation involves connecting one or both of the lateral ventricles with the cisterna magna or the subarachnoid space of the cervical spine. This technique, known as Torkildsen's operation or ventriculo-cisternostomy, was designed for cases of adult hydrocephalus. This type of shunt may successfully drain the excess CSF for many years. Further surgery is usually required in the case of patients with tumours that are causing the obstruction.

CONGENITAL ABNORMALITIES OF THE SPINE

The neural tube is the precursor of the spinal canal (Figure 8.4a). Failure of the neural tube to fuse results in a group of congenital abnormalities commonly described by the term spina bifida.

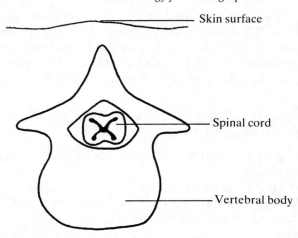

Figure 8.4a   Normal anatomy of the spine

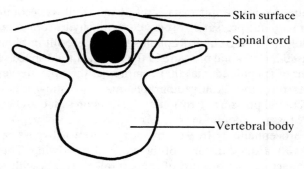

Figure 8.4b   Spina bifida occulta

Spina bifida occulta

In this condition one or a number of the neural arches in the lumbo-sacral region fail to fuse in the midline (Figure 8.4b). This is a common chance radiological finding and usually causes no problems when restricted to isolated vertebrae. If more extensive bony abnormalities are present then this usually indicates that other abnormalities of the spinal cord are also present, e.g. tumours or deformities of the spinal cord. These abnormalities may lead to disruption of normal bladder and bowel function and loss of the ability to walk.

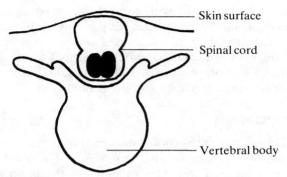

Figure 8.4c   Meningocoele

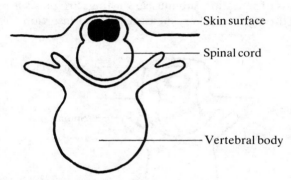

Figure 8.4d   Meningomyelocoele

Meningocoele

This is a common abnormality which consists of herniation of the subarachnoid space through the bony abnormality of the neural arch (Figure 8.4c). The defective area becomes covered with a protective layer of tissue and forms a thin walled sac on the skin surface. This usually causes no neurological abnormalities and is easily removed without further complications.

Meningomyelocoele

This is a much more complex type of meningocoele. The range of bony defects is more extensive and is complicated by herniation of the meninges and spinal cord through the defect (Figure 8.4d). The cord is damaged and the condition is associated with some form of paralysis, disruption to bladder function and hydrocephalus (75 per cent of all cases). Skin closure may be carried out to prevent infection of the cord. A shunt is also inserted to control the hydrocephalus. Despite corrections to the site of the lesion and control of hydrocephalus the child is usually left with some sort of handicap. These include paraplegia and incontinence.

Syringomyelocoele

In this condition the spinal cord is disrupted by a central dilatation of the cord (Figure 8.4e). A cystic area develops that is filled with CSF. The condition is associated with abnormalities of the brain (syringomyelia). Expansion of the cord is thought to develop through anomalies in the posterior fossa forcing CSF into the cystic space. The condition results in gradual loss of sensation and muscle wasting. Prognosis is poor but may be improved through temporary measures such as insertion of shunts.

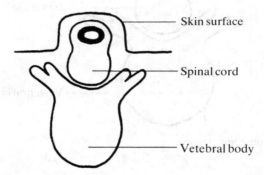

Figure 8.4e   Syringomyelocoele

Fusion of adjacent vertebrae

Occurs most commonly in the cervical spine. It produces shortness of the neck and is known as the Klippel-Feil syndrome. This condition may also be associated with abnormalities of the foramen magnum (platybasia or basilar impression).

The Klippel-Feil abnormality may be associated with a variety of abnormalities including narrowing of the foramen magnum with no symptoms, to paraplegia. Hydrocephalus may be a secondary development, due to obstruction of the fourth ventricle by the abnormal foramen magnum, or by the presence of the cerebellar tonsils within the foramen magnum.

Myelography may demonstrate a complete or partial block of the spinal cord or other spinal abnormalities. CT scanning may show spinal abnormalities and hydrocephalus. The condition is relieved by removing bone from the foramen magnum thereby 'decompressing' the posterior fossa.

Spondylolisthesis

This is a defect in the fusion of the components of a vertebra. This is due to the non-development of the pars interarticularis and usually occurs at the level of L4–5. As a result the vertebral body moves forward producing a step in the spinal column. This may cause symptoms due to pressure on nerve roots and in some cases requires surgery to remove damaged discs and to give stability by fusing the vertebrae.

VASCULAR DISORDERS

Figures 8.5a and 8.5b show the main arteries and veins of the brain.

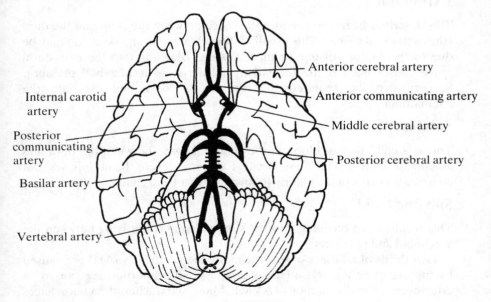

Figure 8.5a   Arteries of the brain (circle of Willis)

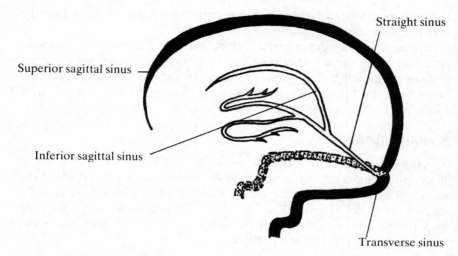

Figure 8.5b   Main venous sinuses of the brain

Intracranial haemorrhage

Extradural

This describes haemorrhage into the space between the skull and the dura (the extradural space). This usually follows trauma to the skull and may be due to the rupture of one or more vessels. Bleeding into the extradural space causes haematoma formation and a rise in intracranial pressure. Surgery may be required to stop the bleeding and evacuate the haematoma.

Subdural

This is a collection of blood in the subdural space between the dura and arachnoid mater. This may occur following severe head injuries but commonly occurs in the elderly following minor head trauma.

Subarachnoid

This results from bleeding into the subarachnoid space lying between the arachnoid and pia mater.

Two-thirds of all cases of subarachnoid haemorrhage (SAH) are caused by rupture of an aneurysm (see p.167), a small proportion are caused by arteriovenous malformations (AVM). Many subarachnoid haemorrhages occur through an unknown cause.

The haemorrhage produces a variety of effects dependent upon the extent. If conscious, the patient may present with a severe headache. The patient may lose consciousness. The condition is also associated with vomiting in the earlier stages, and neck stiffness, which develops later.

In cases of rapid onset of headache, a subarachnoid haemorrhage is suspected and is usually investigated by lumbar puncture and CT scanning. CT scanning may be used as the initial course of investigation in cases with suspected cerebral haematoma where lumbar puncture could complicate the condition.

Bloodstained CSF at lumbar puncture may indicate that a subarachnoid haemorrhage has occurred, although initially the CSF may remain clear. CT scanning may show blood in the ventricles, basal cisterns or Sylvian fissure. The cause of the bleed is usually elucidated by cerebral angiography. If a cerebral aneurysm or AVM is found then surgery is usually carried out to prevent further haemorrhage. Surgery is usually reserved for patients who are conscious and who show positive signs of recovery. Prognosis is usually poor for those patients who lose consciousness following a bleed and are still unconscious some hours later.

Intracerebral (haematoma)

Intracerebral lesions account for a large proportion of deaths each year. The condition is often given the general name of cerebrovascular accident (CVA). CVA covers both haemorrhages within the cerebral substance and vascular insufficiency to the brain (ischaemic strokes or simply 'strokes').

Cerebral

Cerebral haemorrhage is an area of bleeding within the cerebral hemisphere. This is due to a number of causes, including:

(1) Hypertension. This is a frequent cause of cerebral haemorrhage and commonly occurs in the elderly where blood vessels may be prone to rupture due to the presence of atheroma. In these cases the haemorrhage usually occurs in the basal ganglia.
(2) Rupture of intracranial aneurysms. The site of the aneurysm determines the area of brain affected (see p.170).
(3) Arteriovenous malformation. These highly vascular structures may give rise to intracerebral or subarachnoid bleeding.
(4) Trauma. Severe head injuries may cause cerebral haemorrhage.

The haemorrhage produces a variety of effects. The patient may lose consciousness and may remain comatose. Confusion and severe headache are also associated with the condition. Hemiplegia may also develop.

Bleeding may be progressive and is frequently fatal. Approximately 60 per cent of patients who survive cerebral haemorrhages are monoplegic.

CT scanning is the best method to demonstrate the extent of the bleeding. Extensive bleeding may rupture into the ventricles producing bloodstained CSF on lumbar puncture. Cerebral haematomas may be restricted to small areas of brain tissue producing localized effects. Multiple small (punctate) haemorrhages may also be seen scattered throughout the brain tissue. These are usually associated with trauma and are common in boxers. CT scanning is now frequently used on boxers to show the presence and extent of these small lesions.

In cases of extensive bleeding, surgery may be of little help. With cases of localized cerebral bleeding, the evacuation of the haemorrhage may be easily carried out with a good prognosis. Underlying pathology, e.g. aneurysms or arteriovenous malformations, may also be controlled surgically.

Vascular insufficiency

Arterial disease

Vascular insufficiency in the arteries (Plate 7) is due to stenosis or occlusion of the carotid, vertebral or other cerebral arteries. This causes an area of the brain to become poorly oxygenated, which leads to the tissue becoming ischaemic and impairing function. The tissue may become infarcted if the blood supply is restricted for a sufficiently long period.

The carotid arteries have been extensively studied due to their accessibility.

Atheroma usually causes stenosis of the carotid arteries. The internal carotid is most commonly affected. The build up of atheroma may lead to a total block of the artery. Emboli from the left atrium or from myocardial infarcts may also lead to block of the carotids. Atheromatous disease is particularly associated with hypertension.

Severe stenosis or occlusions of the neck and head vessels produces a variety of effects. Stenosis of one carotid vessel may produce little effect due to the distribution of blood within the circle of Willis. Narrowing may produce transient ischaemic attacks (TIAs) which are characterized by episodes of limb weakness, due to micro emboli separating from the block within the artery, and affecting small areas of the brain. These attacks may last for minutes or hours. Larger emboli may cause infarction of areas of the brain tissue ('strokes'). This usually leads to severe loss of limb function or loss of speech, depending upon the area of the brain affected.

When the vertebral or basilar arteries are affected, the patient may

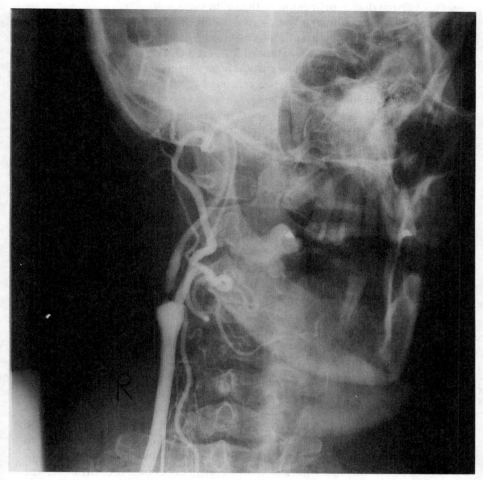

Plate 7   Severe stenosis of the right carotid artery

suffer vertigo due to disruption to the brain stem.

Carotid angiography may be carried out in cases of suspected stenosis or occlusion to show the extent and position of the lesion. CT scanning may be used to demonstrate the extent of infarcted tissue. Doppler and isotope studies may also demonstrate a carotid artery stenosis.

Carotid artery stenosis may be treated by microsurgical techniques to repair the site of the narrowing. In severe cases a bypass may be established around the stenosis or occlusion. Patients who have not suffered from a stroke, but who may have had episodes of TIA, and have had a stenosis demonstrated but do not have multiple vessel disease, are thought to be suitable for surgery.

Intracranial aneurysms

The majority of intractranial aneurysms (Plate 8a & b) are of the saccular type. They develop due to weaknesses in the muscle coat of the arteries and are accentuated by the presence of arteriosclerosis and hypertension. Intracranial aneurysms usually develop on the anterior portion of the circle of Willis. The internal carotid is the most commonly affected. Four main sites lying on the circle are also affected: (1) at the origin of the posterior communicating artery, (2) at the origin of the ophthalmic artery, (3) in the cavernous sinus, and (4) at the terminal bifurcation.

Aneurysms that are most liable to rupture are found on the anterior communicating artery.

In the posterior fossa aneurysms may be found on the basilar and vertebral arteries. Approximately 10 per cent of patients have more than one aneurysm.

Many intracranial aneurysms produce no symptoms. Unruptured aneurysms may produce symptoms when they become large enough to compress surrounding structures. This may occur with some aneurysms that develop on the internal carotid artery behind the orbit. Large aneurysms may compress the optic nerve and in some cases the optic chiasma.

Rupture of an aneurysm causes bleeding which usually shows as blood in the subarachnoid space on CT scanning. Blood may also appear in the CSF due to movement of blood into the ventricles.

The site of the aneurysm is located by CT scanning and angiography. Four vessel angiography is carried out to exclude multiple aneurysms.

A ruptured aneurysm produces infarction of the area of brain supplied by the blood vessels involved. Hydrocephalus may develop following rupture of an aneurysm due to obstruction to the flow of CSF. The patient

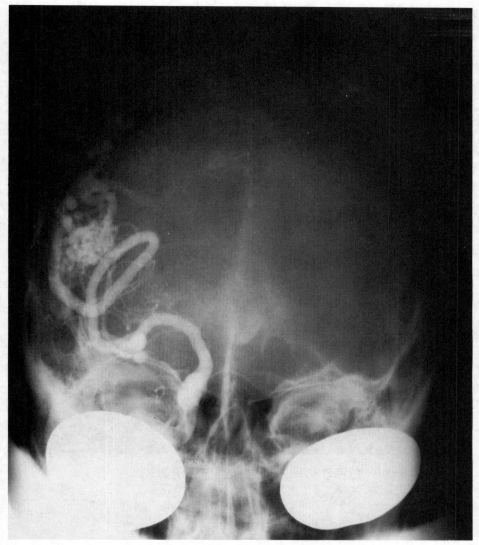

Plate 8a   Arteriovenous malformation (Towne's projection)

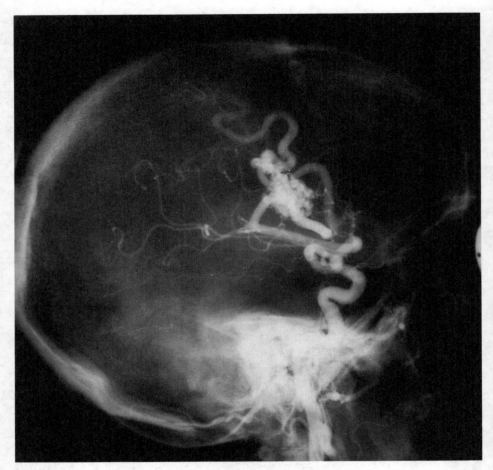

Plate 8b   Arteriovenous malformation (Lateral projection)

may lose consciousness due to disruption of areas of the brain surrounding the ruptured aneurysm.

Initial treatment of a ruptured subarachnoid haemorrhage usually involves rest. Patients with SAH must not sit up, because change in posture may cause changes in the intracranial pressure that may complicate the situation. Following demonstration of the site of bleeding patients may undergo surgery to control the bleeding. A number of techniques are available. The commonest is occlusion of the neck of the aneurysm. This is carried out by isolating the aneurysm from the vessel feeding it. A clip is usually placed on the neck of the aneurysm under control of an operating microscope. This operation carries a number of risks due to disruption of the brain tissue and the possibility of further bleeding. Hemiplegia may result post-operatively. Aneurysms of the anterior communicating artery are the most difficult to clip. Patients with multiple aneurysms may be treated by clipping both leaking and 'silent' aneurysms to prevent further rupture.

Arteriovenous malformation (angioma)

This is a congenital malformation of the blood vessels (Plate 9). The abnormality usually starts as a collection of capillaries that enlarge and rupture to form arteriovenous fistulae. The malformation enlarges due to the force of the arterial blood in the thin-walled veins. This may deprive the brain of portions of its blood supply and produce areas of ischaemia. Angiomas are commonly found in the cerebral hemispheres. These malformations may rupture and cause intracerebral bleeding. The condition may be associated with epilepsy and severe headaches.

CT scanning using contrast media is required to demonstrate the site of the malformation. Angiography follows to show the anatomy of the vessels within the malformation. Angiomas frequently calcify and this may be demonstrated on plain skull radiographs. The condition may be treated by surgical removal of the malformation or embolisation under radiological control.

THE NERVOUS SYSTEM

Infections

Meningitis

Meningitis describes any inflammation of the meninges due to the introduction of foreign organisms. The areas most commonly affected are

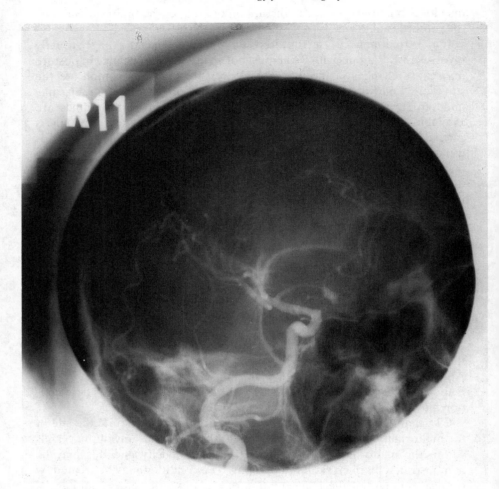

Plate 9   Aneurysm of the anterior communicating artery

the pia and arachnoid membranes, the subarachnoid space and the ventricles. A number of types of meningitis exist: suppurative, tuberculous and meningococcal.

Effects

Meningitis is characterized clinically by severe headache and neck stiffness, due to irritation of the meninges, and may be mistaken for a subarachnoid haemorrhage. In patients with meningitis passive neck flexion is severely limited. Meningitis also damages localized areas of the brain producing cranial nerve palsies.

In infants and young children the signs of meningitis manifest less clearly than in the adult. An enlarged head with expanded fontanelles in the very young may give a clue to the diagnosis. The child may appear irritable and diagnosis is confirmed by lumbar puncture. *Haemophilus influenzae* and *E. coli* are common causes of infantile meningitis.

Suppurative (pyogenic)

Suppurative meningitis is due to infection of the meninges with pyogenic organisms. The organisms most commonly involved are the pneumococci, meningococci, staphylococci and streptococci.

The infection reaches the meninges via a number of routes:

(1) Direct spread from adjacent infections, e.g. the sinuses, cerebral abscess and mastoids. In these cases the infection is often caused by streptococci.
(2) Blood-borne infections spread from other sites. Pneumococcal infections may be spread from the lung to the meninges.
(3) Direct wounds that penetrate directly into the meninges, e.g. fractures, surgery, may cause meningitis to develop.

Suppurative meningitis causes the meninges to become inflamed and a purulent exudate is produced that passes into the subarachnoid space. The infection does not remain localized but has a tendency to spread into the cerebral ventricles. Lumbar puncture performed in cases of suspected purulent meningitis show the CSF to contain organisms with a high content of polymorphonuclear leucocytes (200–3,000 cells per mm^3). Patients who develop suppurative meningitis may have undergone a course of antibiotics to treat other infections. This makes it difficult to culture specific bacteria from the CSF and may mask the symptoms of meningitis.

The condition is treated by the use of antibiotics, e.g. penicillin, ampicillin, given intravenously. In advanced cases the antibiotics may be given directly into the subarachnoid space. If the condition is treated in the early stages there is good resolution and recovery. In untreated cases the risk of mortality is high.

Tuberculous

This is now a rare form of meningitis due to the widespread control of the disease through inoculation. The disease spreads via the blood from the lungs to the subarachnoid space. Miliary tuberculosis more commonly produces tuberculous meningitis. The tuberculosis may develop as a cerebral lesion and spread into the CSF via the ventricles. This may cause obstruction to the flow of CSF with a resultant non-communicating hydrocephalus. The condition is treated by using antibiotics, e.g. strep-tomycin. In advanced cases mortality is high.

Non-suppurative (aseptic)

This type of meningitis is caused by infection of the CSF with non-pyogenic organisms. In general, no organism can be cultured from the CSF. Tuberculous meningitis is often included in this group. Other causes of aspetic meningitis include:

(1) Viruses. Viral meningitis is caused by a variety of viruses including polio virus, mumps and herpes zoster. Viral meningitis usually occurs as part of a more complex disease affecting the central nervous system, e.g. encephalitis.
(2) Syphilis. This is an uncommon cause of meningitis. It is associated with secondary or tertiary syphilis.
(3) Foreign materials. Meningitis may develop due to the presence of chemicals in the CSF. The presence of contrast media in the subarachnoid space following myelography may cause meningitis to develop. This may be termed secondary aseptic meningitis.

Viral infections

Poliomyelitis

Infection due to polio virus is almost eradicated in Great Britain due to the widespread use of vaccination. The disease is infectious and is passed by direct contact or contamination of food and water. The disease follows two stages. Initially the patient shows general systemic symptoms including headache and fever. The disease then progresses and the legs begin to waste and lose muscle tone resulting in paralysis. Mortality is high unless the patient is kept alive on a machine giving assisted respiration.

Viral encephalitis

Viral encephalitis is caused by a number of viruses that act directly on the nerve cells of the brain. The viruses causing encephalitis include polio virus and herpes simplex. Herpes simplex is a virus that produces infections of the skin, particularly around the mouth. However, if the virus invades the brain it produces an acute form of encephalitis (acute necrotizing encephalitis). This is rapidly fatal unless treated.

Viral encephalitis produces inflammation and congestion of the meninges and brain together with multiple small haemorrhages. This leads to degeneration of the nerve cells, particularly in the area of the pons, substantia nigra and medulla. Occasionally, the condition affects the spinal cord (ancephalomyelitis).

In the early stages the patient suffers from pyrexia, headache and increasing confusion. The condition may progress to paralysis and epilepsy.

Unless treated, viral encephalitis has a high mortality rate. In the case of herpes simplex encephalitis accurate diagnosis through CT scanning and biopsy is required to start treatment with antiviral agents. Patients who recover from encephalitis may be left with a variety of disabilities, e.g. Parkinsonism, due to localized destruction of areas of brain tissue.

Herpes zoster

This is caused by the varicella virus, which also causes chicken-pox. In some cases this becomes localized to the dorsal root or cranial nerve ganglia. This gives rise to skin vesicles over the sensory distribution of the affected nerve producing degenerative changes in the nerve and severe pain. The condition is commonly known as 'shingles'.

Intracranial abscess

Intracranial abscess is defined as a suppurative inflammation of the brain tissue. The abscess develops around an area of infection within the brain substance. There is a localized build-up of pus with oedema in the surrounding brain tissue. A thin outer membrane may build up around the affected area. The condition may develop through:

(1) Spread from adjacent areas of infection. Diseases of the ear are the commonest cause of abscess formation. Chronic suppurative otitis media causes erosion of the petrous bone and contiguous spread of infection to the temporal lobe. Acute sinusitis and mastoiditis may also give rise to abscess formation due to osteomyelitis and spread into the brain tissue.

(2) Blood spread. Haematogenous brain abscesses develop through blood-borne infection from other areas of suppurative infection, e.g. lung abscesses.
(3) Trauma. Penetrating wounds to the head may introduce infections directly into the brain or abscesses may develop as a post-operative complication.

The presence of an abscess produces a variety of symptoms ranging from headache and pyrexia in the early stages to disruption to consciousness and loss of function and consciousness. The latter symptoms are as a result of the expansion of the abscess causing compression of localized areas of the brain. Epilepsy may develop with frontal and temporal lobe lesions.

CT scanning is frequently used as the first step in diagnosis of an intracranial abscess. The enhanced CT scan usually shows the abscess as an area of ring enhancement due to the disruption of the blood-brain barrier. Distinction between abscess and tumour may be made through a knowledge of the clinical history of the patient. The scan will also demonstrate any movement of the brain caused by the presence of the abscess and evidence of any hydrocephalus.

If left untreated the abscess will continue to expand and cause further problems. Rupture of the abscess may prove fatal. The abscess is treated by giving the patient antibiotics followed by draining the abscess. Antibiotics may be introduced into the site of the abscess. The effectiveness of the surgery is monitored by CT scanning. In some cases multiple small abscesses may be found. These may be treated by complete excision under antibiotic cover.

Demyelinating diseases

Figure 8.6 shows a generalized diagram of a neurone. In the demyelinating diseases the myelin sheath is destroyed leaving the axon intact.

Multiple sclerosis

Multiple sclerosis primarily affects the white matter of the brain and spinal cord. The peripheral nervous system is unaffected. Other areas affected include dorsal tracts of the spinal cord and the brain stem. The myelin sheath is destroyed in patches along the length of the axon. These areas of destruction are called plaques, and contain reduced numbers of normal cells together with abnormal cells. The course of the myelin sheath destruction follows no standard pattern.

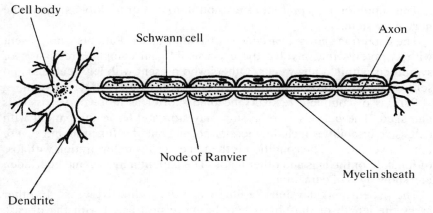

Figure 8.6 A neurone

Causes

The cause or causes of multiple sclerosis are still unknown. Possible causes include viral infections, defects in the immune system, poisons and allergies.

Incidence

The disease occurs in approximately 50 people per 10,000. The disease is most commonly seen in young adults with a mean age of about thirty years. Infrequent cases are seen in the elderly and the very young.

Symptoms and course

Due to the variable incidence and distribution of plaques the presenting symptoms of the disease are varied. Presenting symptoms include muscle weakness, sensory loss and disruption of vision.

Visual loss may vary from slight blurring to blindness. This is due to demyelination of various groups of fibres within the optic nerve. Visual defects may only occur in one eye and in some cases there may be a return to normal sight within a few weeks of onset. This pattern of onset of disease followed by periods of remission is a characteristic of multiple sclerosis.

In some cases weakness of the legs may be the first symptom the patient is aware of. Other patients may present with sensory disturbances such as pins and needles in their legs. Occasionally the disease may present as an acute onset of paraplegia.

The condition may present as disruption to one or multiple areas of the nervous system.

The condition shows a variable course after onset. Patients who present with symptoms that involve the eye usually gain complete remission of symptoms within a few weeks. Others who present with leg weakness and sensory signs may not show full recovery and only gain partial remission.

Periods of complete recovery become shorter as more nerve tissue is damaged. The periods of remission may stop and leave the patient with extensive disabilities including loss of normal bladder function and severe muscle weakness. The condition is then one of slow deterioration with loss of function of the legs and other limbs. The patient may become bedridden and show signs of dementia.

The patient may develop the illness and die within five years. In other cases the length of the illness may be more protracted with the disease lasting for 15–25 years.

Some benign forms of the disease may allow the patient to live with very minor disabilities.

Disabilities caused by the disease may lead to further complications, e.g. pneumonia, bedsores.

Diagnosis

The disease may be diagnosed from its characteristic pattern of onset and remission. Testing for the disease by taking samples of CSF is usually carried out. Magnetic resonance imaging can also be a useful technique to screen for the disease.

Other rarer forms of demyelinating disease exist, such as post-infective encephalomyelitis, which may follow smallpox or measles and cause areas of demyelination due to an autoimmune response in the CNS.

The basal ganglia

The basal ganglia play a major role in the control and co-ordination of movements, initiating and relaying commands from the higher centres to the motor neurones of the spinal cord. Disruption to the basal ganglia produces a number of disorders of co-ordination and movement.

Parkinson's disease (paralysis agitans)

Parkinson's disease is common in the age group 50–70 and is more common in men than women. In other age groups the illness may be caused by encephalitis (post-encephalitic Parkinsonism).

Causes

The causes of Parkinsonism are not fully understood. There is no known genetic link. The disease is thought to be caused by contact with certain chemicals that accelerate the loss of nerve cells in certain parts of the brain. Examination of the affected brain shows loss of nerve cells in the area of the substantia nigra, caudate nucleus and globus pallidus.

Course and symptoms

The first symptoms of Parkinson's disease is usually tremor. The hand may shake very slowly at first but this usually progresses to a constant uncontrolled movement of the hand. This may be accompanied by movement of the head and jaw and rhythmic movements of the thumb and index finger. The disease progresses to dyskinesia which is a disruption of normal voluntary movement. The patient becomes unable to move properly. Movement slows and the patient may frequently fall over. The disease is also associated with increasing rigidity of the muscles with changes of posture while moving. Mental function may remain unchanged, but dementia may be associated with the condition. Speech may also be affected becoming slower and confused. In chronic cases the patient may be left totally immobile with the smallest movement involving immense efforts.

Diagnosis

Screening for the condition is now thought possible using positron emission tomography (PET).

Treatment

Drugs may be used to control the effects of the condition. Patients with Parkinson's disease have a lack of dopamine in the basal ganglia. Increasing the levels of dopamine in the form of levodopa, which is absorbed by the brain, helps the symptoms of the condition. This has side-effects and produces its own involuntary movements. Research is being carried out to synthesize drugs that have the benefits of levodopa without the side-effects.

Huntington's chorea

Chorea is a general term used to describe short involuntary movements without any purpose. The movements occur randomly. Huntington's chorea is a rare hereditary disease transmitted by dominant inheritance. The condition appears in the fifth decade and is latent in the child. The condition is caused by atrophy of the cerebral cortex and basal ganglia, particularly the caudate nucleus. The brain tissue suffers from extensive loss of nerve cells.

The exaggerated involuntary movements of the condition become progressively worse. The patient suffers dementia and complete mental and physical disability. The condition usually ends in premature death. There is no clear way of detecting the disease before it occurs or for treating the condition.

The spinal cord

Motor neurone disease

A degenerative disease of the spinal cord with an unknown cause. Motor neurone disease is a group term that covers three individual conditions of the spinal cord and brain. These include:

(1) Progressive muscular atrophy.
(2) Amyotrophyic lateral sclerosis.
(3) Progressive bulbar palsy.

These conditions produce loss of upper and lower motor neurone function and also affect the cranial nerves of the brain stem.

The condition usually occurs in the age group 35–50. The disease may present by causing muscle wasting of the hands and limbs. If the disease first manifests itself in the progressive bulbar form, then the medulla is first affected and causes difficulties in speech and swallowing. The tongue becomes wasted and it becomes difficult to swallow food.

The disease is progressive and few patients survive more than three years after the onset of the condition. The muscles become progressively wasted and the patient loses weight and may contract pneumonias and an inability to cough properly due to the lengthy periods spent in bed.

The condition is usually treated palliatively by simply making the patient comfortable and giving drugs that may alleviate pain from other conditions resulting from the disease, e.g. bedsores.

Compression of the spinal cord

Compression of the spinal cord may result from:

(1) Crush fractures to the spine.
(2) Prolapsed intervertebral disc caused by rupture of the annulus fibrosus due to strains placed upon the spine. The disc tends to prolapse laterally or posteriorly. This causes compression of the cord, or entrapment of the nerves leaving the cord. Nerve entrapment common-

ly occurs in the lumbar region causing nerve compression (sciatica).

Prolapse also frequently occurs at the level of the seventh cervical vertebra producing cervical root compression. This causes the characteristic parathesia.

(3) Tumours, e.g. neurofibromas, myelomas.
(4) Other disease affecting the bones, e.g. Paget's, tuberculosis, osteoporosis.

These all cause disruption to the spinal cord which leads to ischaemia at the affected site of the cord. In extreme cases this produces loss of motor and sensory functions. The level of compression will determine the extent and type of disturbance caused. Paraplegia and loss of bladder function are common causes of cord compression.

The peripheral nerves

Trauma

Severing of the peripheral nerves is a common form of peripheral nerve disease. This is generally due to trauma. Severing of a peripheral nerve results in immediate loss of conduction in the nerve. Following disruption the distal portion of the nerve may respond to electrical stimulation due to the presence of axoplasm. After a few days the neurones are no longer protected by the axoplasm and the axon rapidly degenerates (Wallerian degeneration). The peripheral neurones recover only if the axis cylinders regenerate. Proper alignment of the two portions of the nerve following trauma will allow the nerve to reform unlike nervous tissue of the CNS.

Peripheral neuropathy

Peripheral neuropathy is a complex condition that usually presents with impairment of sensory function. The patient complains of parathesia. The patient also suffers from muscle weakness and loss of reflexes. Some form of demyelination is associated with peripheral neuropathy.

Causes

There are many causes for peripheral neuropathy, including:

(1) Diabetes and other metabolic diseases.
(2) Alcohol.
(3) Carcinomas.
(4) Connective tissue disease, e.g. polyarteritis nodosa and rheumatoid arthritis.
(5) Toxins, e.g. heavy metals, organic solvents.

(6) The Guillain-Barre syndrome (Landry's paralysis). This may occur at any age with rapid onset and is thought to be due to a type of immunological reaction that affects the peripheral nerves causing demyelination of the neurones.

Tingling of the limbs is noted at first and this is followed by a rapid loss of motor functions. The result is severe paralysis. Respiration is also affected and may result in respiratory paralysis requiring assisted respiration. This is due to the effect of the disease on the cranial nerves.

Prognosis is good and many patients show full recovery provided adequate respiratory support is given.

Peripheral neuropathy is controlled by treating the underlying cause of the illness, e.g. giving insulin and/or controlling diet in diabetics, stopping alcohol intake, etc. Regeneration of nerves occurs in most cases although some patients may be left with minor disabilities.

Tumours

Tissue of the nervous system is divided into nervous and connective or neuroglial types. The connective tissue is broadly composed of:

(1) Astrocytes.
(2) Oligodendrocytes.
(3) Microglial cells.

Gliomas

The gliomas arise from the neuroglia and are named according to the type of neuroglial tissue from which they arise. This classification may vary between the specialists who classify them.

Astrocytoma

This is the commonest type of glioma accounting for approximately 75 per cent of all gliomas. They occur most often in adults but may also occur in children (fibrillary astrocytoma) and are mostly composed of cells similar to astrocytes. Astrocytomas are usually subdivided into four grades of malignancy:

Grade I (fibrillary astrocytoma). This is the least malignant form with the best prognosis. The cells within the tumour closely resemble astrocyte cells, the cells are fairly regular with no signs of anaplasia. This may be classed as a benign form of glioma.

Grade II (astroblastoma). In this category of astrocytoma there is a slight variation in the shape of the astrocyte. The cells begin to show minor abnormalities.

Grade III. This type shows a more extreme abnormality. The tumours contain very few cells that are recognizable as astrocytes.

Grade IV. These may be anaplastic and are the most malignant.

Grades III and IV account for over half of all gliomas.

The above division of tumour types shows the four major groups of gliomas, but a more subtle analysis of tumour type is usually made by considering many factors, e.g. number of cells present in the mass, the rate of mitosis and the presence of haemorrhage. The tumours have a complicated histology and when biopsied may appear as any of the four categories depending upon the site of the biopsy.

The tumours usually occur in the cerebellar hemispheres in adults. They may invade locally or spread across the brain surface. The tumour appears to invade diffusely surrounding tissue and may grow to occupy large areas of tissue.

Ependymoma

This type of glioma arises from tissues of ependymal origin. The tumours arise from tissues lining the ventricles and the central canal of the spinal cord, commonly occurring in the fourth ventricle causing severe obstruction to CSF flow and making removal very difficult. Ependymomas commonly occur in young adults and children. In children the tumour usually begins to grow in the cerebellum. The tumours are grade I-IV with increasing types of malignancy. Some types show as calcified masses on skull radiographs.

Oligodendroglioma

This is a slow-growing tumour found mainly in adults and accounts for approximately 5 per cent of all gliomas. It occurs in the cerebral hemispheres and spreads locally. The tumour may spread via the CSF to other sites. They frequently show areas of calcification and are therefore visible on radiographs.

Treatment of gliomas

Treatment is usually by surgical removal of the glioma. This may involve removal of part or whole of a lobe. Post-operative radiotherapy to the site of the tumour may also be given. Success of the operation and survival depend upon the site and grade of the tumour and age of the patient. Prognosis is usually poor for the higher grades of tumour.

Medulloblastoma

This tumour commonly occurs in children and is more frequent in boys than girls (2:1). Medulloblastomas are tumours of undifferentiated primitive cells which are residual cells of the fetus. Some authorities class medulloblastomas as gliomas. The tumour is highly malignant and grows from the vermis of the cerebellum into the fourth ventricle causing hydrocephalus. Due to spread of the tumour via the CSF, insertion of a shunt will complicate the condition.

This type of tumour is very sensitive to radiation and total irradiation of the brain and spinal cord is carried out. Removal of the tumour may also be attempted. However, despite the use of radiation prognosis is poor due to both seeding of the tumour into the CSF and rapid tumour growth.

Meningioma

This type of tumour arises from the meninges and accounts for approximately 20 per cent of all tumours of the CNS. The tumours most commonly occur in adults. The tumours have a variable appearance, some being rounded like golf balls (global) and some appearing as flat structures *en plaque.*

They occur at many sites, including the falx cerebri, petrous bone, sphenoidal ridge, olfactory groove. Meningiomas are frequently associated with the dura of the skull vault and may occur post-injury. The tumours are attached to the meninges and cause compression of the brain by their slow growth. This may produce bony erosion and compression of surrounding structures. They are rarely malignant but must be removed to prevent damage to nerve centres because of their pressure effect.

Meningiomas are frequently fed by a number of blood vessels. This makes removal of the tumour complicated due to the risk of haemorrhage.

Secondary brain tumours

Secondary brain tumours are more common than primary brain tumours. Most frequent is lung and breast cancer.

Nerve cell

Tumours of nerve cells within the CNS are uncommon. Tumours of the peripheral nervous system are more common.

Neurofibroma

This is a benign tumour of the peripheral nerves. These commonly occur on the cranial nerves and dorsal and posterior spinal roots. The tumours may occur singly or as multiple lesions along the nerve and may grow large enough to cause compression of the nerves and spinal cord. Neurofibromas have a poor acellular structure and appear as a swelling on the nerve. A very small proportion become malignant (neurofibrosarcoma).

Neurofibromatosis

This is a dominant inherited defect that produces a variety of changes in the body. The peripheral nerves are ensheathed with numerous neurofibromas and the skin has areas of brown pigment called *café-au-lait* spots. The condition may also affect the bones and spinal column. The condition may become complicated due to spinal cord compression. Neurofibromas are thought to arise from the Schwann cells.

Embryoplastic

These are rare tumours of the nervous system and include tumours of the pineal gland (pinealomas) and craniopharyngiomas that arise from a remnant of the primitive pharyngeal pouch. Craniopharyngiomas are more common in children.

Epilepsy

An epileptic fit is defined as a brief disorder of cerebral function, usually associated with a disturbance to consciousness and accompanied by an excessive electrical discharge of the cerebral neurones. There are many types of epilepsy. Two broad groups are recognized:

(1) Generalized seizures with loss of consciousness.
(2) Partial or focal fits with no loss of consciousness.

Generalized

There are two common varieties:

Grand mal

A grand mal fit is divided into a number of stages:

(1) Prodromal. This vague preliminary phase may last hours or days and warns the patient of an impending attack.
(2) Aura. This precedes the fit and the patient may experience disturbances to smell or vision.
(3) Tonic stage. The patient loses consciousness and has a spasm of all muscles. The patient may suffer a respiratory arrest. This phase lasts approximately thirty seconds.

(4) Clonic phase. The patient gives powerful jerking movements and at this stage may bite their tongue.

(5) Relaxation. The patient passes into a quiet phase which usually results in normal sleep.

On waking the patient may experience a headache and will probably be confused.

Petit mal

In this type of fit the patient usually suffers from a transient loss of consciousness. The patient interrupts whatever they are doing and loses concentration. These periods of blankness last approximately 15–20 seconds.

Partial or focal

The appearance and events associated with focal epilepsy vary widely and depend upon the area of the brain that is affected.

Temporal lobe

This is the most common site of focal epilepsy. The patient may experience an aura and feeling of *déjà vu*. Consciousness may be retained, although the patient may lose control of motor actions.

Jacksonian

Jacksonian fits are usually confined to one limb. The limb carries out gross involuntary movements. Following the fit the affected limb may be left paralysed.

Diagnosis

CT scanning and radiography are usually carried out to detect underlying lesions that may prompt the fits.

Treatment

Anticonvulsant drugs, e.g. phenobarbitone may be used to control the fits. Removal of stimuli that may prompt fits, e.g. flickering lights, is essential.

THE EAR

The basic structure of the ear can be seen in Figure 8.7.

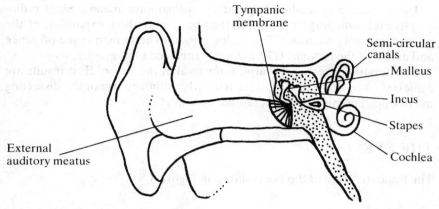

Figure 8.7   Structure of the ear

Otitis media

This is a non-specific infection of the middle ear and may be caused by staphylococci and streptococci. The condition is associated with infections of the upper respiratory tract. Infection is spread from the throat to the ear via the pharyngotympanic tube. The ear becomes filled with pus that may cause perforation of the ear-drum and destruction of the ossicles. Unless controlled with antibiotics or drained the condition becomes chronic. This can lead to further complications including intracranial abscesses or infections of the inner ear (labyrinthitis).

Menière's disease

It is thought that this is caused by an increase in pressure in the endolymph that gives rise to dilatation of the endolymphatic system. This leads to destruction of the hair cells of the organ of Corti. The patient experiences dizziness, vomiting and tinnitus. Microsurgery may be carried out to drain the endolymph and reduce the pressure within the system.

The Acoustic neuroma

This benign tumour arises from the vestibular division of the eighth cranial nerve. This takes place just inside the internal auditory meatus. The tumour grows very slowly compressing the brain and causing bony erosions. It grows into the midbrain and the pons causing a variety of effects including loss of hearing, tinnitus, vomiting, vertigo and raised intracranial pressure.

The condition is readily detected by radiographic means. Skull radiographs and tomography of the petrous bone may show expansion of the internal auditory meatus. CT scanning is used to demonstrate the presence and extent of the tumour. CT has largely replaced tomography.

The tumour is treated by surgical removal of the lesion. Best results are achieved when the tumour is detected early, although use of the dissecting microscope has made removal far more complete.

THE EYE

The basic structure of the eye is shown in Figure 8.8.

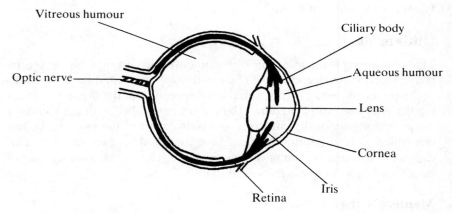

Figure 8.8   Structure of the eye

Cataract

This is an opacity of the lens.

Congenital

This may be transmitted as a autosomal dominant condition or it may be associated with an episode of rubella (German measles) during pregnancy. Contracting German measles, particularly within the first few months of pregnancy, causes a higher incidence of congenital abnormalities of the eye and heart. Immunization against rubella has now reduced the risk to the baby, although due to recent scares over the vaccines used the incidence of rubella may increase again.

Senile

This is an increased sclerosis of the lens. The fibres at the centre of the lens become thickened and cause an opacity to build up (nuclear cataract). In some cases the outer part of the lens may opacify (cortical cataract). Cataracts may also occur in long-term diabetes.

Traumatic

Penetrating injuries of the eye may cause disruption to the lens. As the lens heals fibres may cover the lens and make it opaque.

Radiation

Repeated exposure to ionizing radiation may cause cataracts to form.

Glaucoma

An increase of intra-ocular tension due to poor drainage of aqueous humour from the eye. This may be due to trauma to the eye, congenital defects or infections. If uncorrected it may lead to atrophy of the retina, ciliary body and the iris. Cataract formation may also occur.

Papilloedema

This is an oedema of the optic disc caused by raised intracranial pressure due to the presence of tumours and other space-occupying lesions. The condition may also be associated with hypertension. Papilloedema may be one of the first signs of an intracranial tumour and unless corrected can lead to visual failure. The optic disc appears swollen and as the condition progresses it brings about optic nerve atrophy and blindness.

Tumours

Retinoblastoma

This is a congenital tumour of the eye that is detected in children at approximately eighteen months. It is an hereditary condition and may occur bilaterally. The tumour spreads over the retina and may spread into the brain via the optic nerve. The tumour is not pigmented and gives an opaque white appearance to the eye. The child develops glaucoma. The tumour may metastasise to bone.

The tumour is treated by removal of the eye (enucleation) and/or radiotherapy with good results in early treatment. Sight is frequently preserved. Genetic counselling is given to families with known history of retinoblastomas.

Malignant melanoma

This is the most common malignant tumour of the eye and may start to grow from the iris, ciliary body or the choroid. The tumour invades the eye and disrupts the retina. Pigmentation increases with malignancy. Heavy pigmentation is thought to carry a poor prognosis.

Two types of melanoma are recognized and are classified by their histology: spindle cell type and epithelioid. The latter is considered more malignant.

In advanced cases the eye may be removed. Other cases may be treated by radiotherapy. Prognosis is better for melanomas of the iris.

Glioma

Gliomas may affect the optic nerve anywhere along its length.

9

SKIN, CONNECTIVE TISSUE AND MUSCLE DISEASES

THE SKIN

The skin is divided into two layers, the outer epidermis and the inner dermis. Lying beneath the dermis is the subcutaneous layer.

The epidermis is composed of keratinizing stratified squamous epithelium. This complex connective tissue is subdivided into an outer horny layer and an inner germinative zone. The outer horny layer is continuously renewed by cells from the germinative zone. A more detailed structure is shown in Figure 9.1.

The colour of the skin is determined by a number of elements. Melanocytes lying within the basal cell layer of the germinative zone secrete melanin, a brown pigment. This is confined to the skin, choroid of the eye, the adrenals and the meninges. The secretion of melanin is controlled by a melanin-stimulating hormone released by the pituitary gland.

In the keratinized area of the horny zone is found keratin, a yellow-orange pigment that also helps to colour the skin.

Further skin coloration is added by oxyhaemoglobin and carboxy-haemoglobin travelling through the fine network of vessels within the skin surface. Complete absence of skin pigment is called albinism and is a recessive Mendelian characteristic. In cases of albinism the skin is coloured only by the blood running through the blood vessels beneath the skin surface.

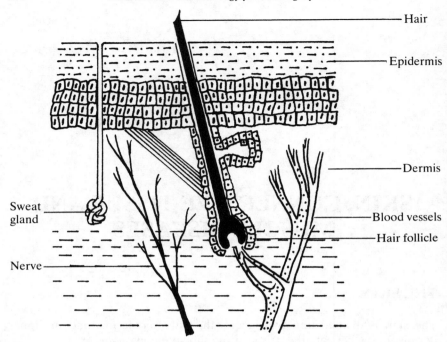

Figure 9.1 Structure of the skin

Inflammations

Eczema

This is an inflammatory reaction of the skin. It is usually caused by an allergic reaction to a specific substance. In the acute form contact with a substance causes a localized skin reaction (dermatitis). This becomes more generalized as the reaction spreads causing an area of rash composed of small blisters or vesicles.

In chronic eczema the changes are more dramatic. The skin is greatly thickened (hyperkeratosis) and becomes inflamed and scaly. The skin is easily removed and is painful and inflamed.

The condition is controlled by isolating the cause of the underlying skin reaction.

Acne vulgaris

This common condition is frequently found in adolescents and is thought to be caused by the presence and levels of certain hormones in the body. For example, it is known that androgens cause hypertrophy of the sebaceous glands, the basic underlying cause of acne.

Enlargement of the sebaceous gland causes them to fail to drain properly. This leads to secondary infections of the gland and disruption of the hair follicle. The condition is characterized by periods of infection followed by intervals of remission. This can produce scarring of the epidermis.

Tumours

Benign

Warts

These benign skin lesions are probably caused by virus infections. They may be spread by direct contact. The skin becomes inflamed and shows hyperkeratosis. A number of types of this benign lesion are recognized:

(1) Verruca vulgaris. This is the common wart.
(2) Verruca plantaris. This commonly occurs on the sole of the foot. Pressure applied to the foot spreads the infection over a wider area.
(3) Condyloma acuminata. These are also called venereal warts and are found in the ano-genital region.

Malignant

Malignant skin cancers occur more commonly in countries with a predominantly white population. Skin cancers are more common among the 60–80 year age group and most frequently occur on the skin of the face.

Causes

(1) Sunlight/UV. Prolonged exposure to sunlight is known to cause skin cancers. The skin becomes inflamed and dries producing areas of pigmented hyperkeratotic skin. Skin cancers develop from these areas. The skin is usually protected by the skin pigments, e.g. melanin. In white Australians skin cancers account for almost 50 per cent of all cancers. This high incidence is due to a lack of protective pigmentation which is present in native Australians. Skin cancer, as expected, is much higher in albinos where no protection to sunlight is given due to the absence of skin pigments.
(2) Chemicals. Prolonged exposure to some hydrocarbons, e.g. creosote, may cause skin cancers. Arsenic is also known to produce skin cancers.
(3) Exposure to ionizing radiation. Skin cancers may occur following therapeutic treatment using radiation. Radiation workers also have a

higher risk of developing skin cancers.
(4) Underlying disease. Long-standing scars following burns and trauma
    or extensive ulceration may be complicated by skin cancers.

Types

The two commonest types of skin cancer are:

(1) Basal cell (rodent ulcer). This occurs more commonly than the
    squamous cell type and is a very slow-growing lesion. The tumour is
    composed of closely packed cells and usually occurs as a raised, ulcer-
    ated area of skin. Basal cell carcinomas usually spread by direct inva-
    sion. As the lesion commonly occurs on the face this produces invasion
    of the paranasal sinuses, the nasal cavity and the cranial cavity. Metas-
    tases to blood and lymph are rare.
(2) Squamous cell. The appearances of squamous cell carcinoma is more
    variable than the basal cell type. The tumour may appear as an
    elevated portion of ulcerated tissue or as a crater in the skin surface.
    All types usually show areas of keratin formation. The tumour spreads
    by local invasion, although the rate of spread is highly variable. Later
    lymphatic spread does occur, but blood-borne metastases are un-
    common.

Classification

The extent of the skin cancer may be graded using the international TNM
classification of malignant cancers:

T is skin cancer *in situ*.
T1 is a superficial cancer measuring 2 cm or less.
T2 is a tumour measuring 2–5 cm and showing a limited invasion of
    surrounding tissue.
T3 indicates a tumour over 5 cm that has invaded the dermis.
T4 is the most extensive form and indicates invasion of other structures and
    tissues, e.g. cartilage and bone.

Treatment

Treatment of both types of cancer is by surgery and radiotherapy.
Radiotherapy is generally used on the less invasive types (T1 and T2).
Surgery is used on more advanced cases with invasion of adjacent
structures. Removal of large areas of tissue may be necessary with the use
of reconstructive surgery and skin grafting. Techniques have been
improved by the use of lasers which allow more accurate removal of
tumours.

Prognosis

With efficient early treatment, the prognosis is good for both types of cancer. The five-year survival rate for squamous cell carcinomas is approximately 95 per cent.

Malignant melanoma

This is an uncommon tumour. It occurs most frequently in Australia and New Zealand where it accounts for 5–6 deaths per 100,000. The lesion may grow on any portion of the body, but more commonly occurs on the lower limbs, feet and neck. Malignant melanomas most commonly occur in adults.

Causes

Over 50 per cent of all malignant melanomas arise from a pre-existing, benign, pigmented lesion, e.g. the intradermal naevus cell (mole). The naevus is usually superficial and is stained brown by the presence of melanin. When a malignant melanoma develops, the patient usually reports a deepening of the colour of the naevus, an increase in its size or bleeding at the site of the naevus. If a melanoma is suspected diagnosis is confirmed by biopsy of the lesion.

In some cases the melanoma may arise from unaffected skin tissue. In these cases the tumour grows from melanocytes of the basal layer of the epidermis. In approximately 15 per cent of all cases the melanoma contains no pigment (achromic melanoma).

Spread

Malignant melanomas are fast-growing tumours. The malignant phase of growth is usually preceded by a pre-malignant period. This may last for many years.

Once a malignant change takes place growth is rapid. Direct invasion of surrounding tissue takes place with extension of the area of pigmentation and the spread of satellite lesions around the area of the primary focus. Early spread to regional lymph nodes may also be noted. Blood-borne spread may also occur early in the disease with secondary spread to the lungs, brain and liver. However, spread may occur to any organ.

In some cases there may be a spontaneous regression of the primary tumour while the secondary deposits continue to grow.

The tumour may be staged by the depth to which it has infiltrated the skin (Breslow's classification).

Treatment

Surgical removal of the melanoma is carried out together with excision of an area of tissue around the site of the lesion. This also includes removal of a layer of subcutaneous fat and muscle fascia to exclude local invasion. This usually requires the use of skin grafts to cover the site of surgery. Excision of local lymph nodes may also be carried out. Radiotherapy may also be given to treat the melanoma. Chemotherapy is usually used to treat localized areas of invasion.

Prognosis

Prognosis of the melanoma relies upon the depth to which the lesion has penetrated and the extent of invasion to lymph nodes. Early diagnosis is essential. With surgical removal of the tumour and the absence of regional metastases there is a five-year survival rate of approximately 60 per cent. Most fatal cases result from widespread secondary spread. Recurrence of the lesion may occur many years after removal of the primary lesion.

Kaposi's sarcoma

This is a rare tumour that affects the skin and arises from the blood vessels within the skin. The skin becomes infiltrated with a variety of cells, e.g. lymphocytes and plasma cells. The condition is usually benign. In approximately 10 per cent of cases there is a widespread loss of vascularity with fatal results. This type of tumour also affects patients with the acquired immune deficiency syndrome (AIDS) or human immunodeficiency virus (HIV).

CONNECTIVE TISSUE

Connective tissues (Figure 9.2) have many functions in the body, both structural and defensive. Connective tissues are widely distributed and may be divided into basic connective tissue and special connective tissue, e.g. cartilage and bone.

Connective tissues are composed of a matrix within which are suspended a collection of cells. The matrix is further composed of a ground substance and a fibrous element. The fibrous element is composed mainly of white collagen fibres. The matrix is formed from a suspension of carbohydrates.

The cellular elements of connective tissue include:

(1) Fibroblasts. These produce the collagen element of the matrix. Fibroblasts are also active in wound repair. Fibroblast activity is

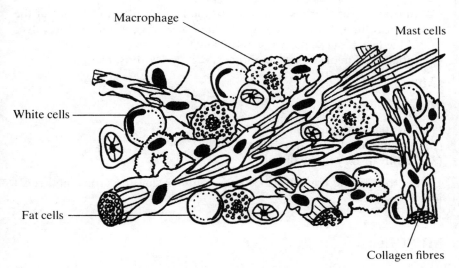

Figure 9.2   Connective tissue showing variety of cells and loose structure

influenced by factors such as diet, the level of vitamin C and steroid hormones in the body.

(2) Lymphocytes and plasma cells. These produce large amounts of antibodies.
(3) Macrophages. These have a phagocytic action and are capable of ingesting and destroying foreign material.
(4) Mast cells are involved in the inflammatory reaction to injury. When disrupted they release histamine. This gives the itching associated with allergic reactions.
(5) Fat cells.

Basic connective tissues exist in two main forms: irregular (loose sheets of tissue) and regular (ligaments and tendons).

Systemic lupus erythematosus (SLE)

This is a disease producing widespread effects. The condition produces changes in the structure of connective tissues, often with the loss of collagen fibres. These changes produce:

(1) Skin rashes.
(2) Rheumatoid arthritis.
(3) Breakdown of the walls of arteries with necrotic changes (necrotizing arteritis).

(4) In some cases there is a necrosis of the heart wall with rupture of the endocardium. This leads to the formation of vegetations on the valves of the heart, particularly the mitral and tricuspid valves.

(5) Inflammation of serous membranes, e.g. pericarditis, pleurisy.

Causes

These include:

(1) Possible viral infection.
(2) Production of auto-antibodies.
(3) Family history of the disease.

Unless treated the condition becomes complex due to cardiac and renal involvement.

MUSCLE

Skeletal or striated muscle (Figure 9.3) is composed of long, cylindrical fibres. Each of these fibres is a specialized cell bounded by a plasma membrane called the sarcolemma. This encloses the cytoplasm of the fibre, called the sarcoplasm. The sarcoplasm contains peripherally placed nuclei and a cytoplasm divided into myofibrils that extend the length of the fibre. On staining these fibres show cross-banding or striations. Individual fibres are bound together by reticular fibres forming the endomysium. Groups of fibres are bound into groups called fasiculi by connective tissues, mainly composed of collagen. This tissue is known as the perimysium. Many fasiculi are bound together into the muscle by the epimysium. The

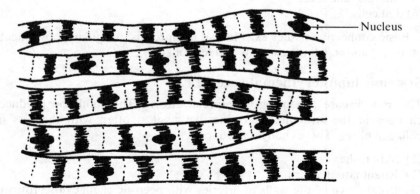

Figure 9.3 Structure of striated muscle

connective tissue layers run throughout and around the muscle fibres helping to support the fibres and supply the muscles with blood vessels and nerves.

Skeletal muscle is innervated by myelinated motor neurones.

Myasthenia gravis

This is a disease characterized by muscle weakness that is usually increased on exertion.

In myasthenia gravis there has been shown to be a lack of the neurotransmitter acetyl choline. This is thought to be due to an anti-striated antibody that has been isolated from the blood of some myasthenic patients.

Approximately 10–20 per cent of cases are associated with a thymoma, or, in younger cases, thymic hyperplasia. Anti-striated antibody is frequently isolated from the blood of patients with thymoma. It is thought that the thymus stimulates the production of anti-striated muscle antibody. Measuring the level of this antibody in the blood can be used in the diagnosis of thymoma. The thymus also produces a number of immunological disruptions. Removal of the thymus frequently produces improvement of the condition.

Muscular dystrophies

The muscular dystrophies are a group of rare inherited diseases of muscle that are characterized by progressive muscular weakness. The specific cause of the disease is still unknown. The disease produces changes mainly in striated muscle tissue. In early stages of the disease there is evidence of loss of muscle fibres and areas of necrosis. As the condition progresses there is replacement of the muscle tissue with fibrous connective tissue and fat. In some cases the cardiac muscle may also be affected.

A number of types of the disease have been described, all characterized by weakness:

(1) Duchenne type. This is an X-linked recessive form of the disease and therefore usually only occurs in males. Symptoms usually occur after the first year of life when the child begins to walk. The child frequently falls and has difficulty in walking. The trunk muscles and arms also begin to weaken as the child becomes older. The child develops a scoliosis and by adolescence is usually unable to walk. The condition becomes worse as respiration becomes affected. Respiration is shallow and the patient is affected by numerous episodes of chest infection. These usually prove fatal by the third decade.

(2) Becker dystrophy. This is also an X-linked disease and presents in a similar way to the Duchenne type, but with slower onset. The child develops symptoms in late childhood or early adolescence.

(3) Other types. Other specific types of muscular dystrophy affecting both males and females are also described, e.g. facioscapulohumeral dystrophy.

There is no specific treatment for muscular dystrophy. Supportive treatment may be given, e.g. splints and braces to support severely weakened limbs. Genetic counselling is given to families with affected children.

Muscular atrophy

This is loss of the muscle bulk, the muscle becoming smaller due to, e.g. disuse following injury. In extreme cases the muscle becomes replaced by fibrous tissue.

10
DISEASES OF THE URINO-GENITAL SYSTEM

THE KIDNEY

Figure 10.1 shows the basic anatomy while Figure 10.2 shows the basic functional unit of the kidney, the nephron. Each of these units consist of a blind-ended tube and is divided into:

(1) The glomerulus, which acts as a very fine filter.
(2) The proximal tubule, which reabsorbs water from the glomerular filtrate.
(3) The loop of Henle, which reabsorbs salt and water.
(4) The distal tubule, which helps control pH balance.
(5) The collecting tubule, which collects the urine formed in the nephron and empties into a calyx.

The major part of the nephron is confined to the cortex of the kidney.

Measurement of renal length

The longitudinal length is the most commonly used dimension in assessing the current state of the kidneys. The adult kidney measures between 10 and 16 cm along its longitudinal axis. The length is variable with age and is greatest in the young adult. The two kidneys are usually of very similar lengths. A difference in length of no greater than 1.5 cm is considered to be within normal limits. A chart of normal kidney size and expected normal variations has been compiled.

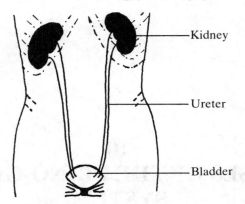

Figure 10.1   Basic anatomy of the urinary tract

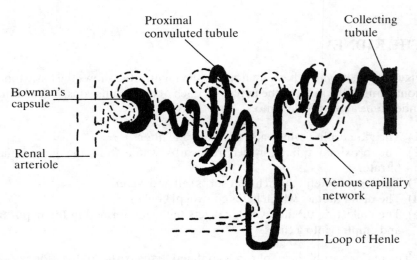

Figure 10.2   Structure of the nephron

Hydronephrosis

This is dilation of the renal pelvis and calyces. This is due to slow progressive obstruction at any level of the urinary tract as the result of the presence of calculi or clots within the lumen of the ureter, strictures of the ureter or gravid uterus. If long-standing, the condition may lead to renal failure.

Proteinuria

Protein in the urine may be caused by:

(1) Glomerulonephritis.
(2) Renal infections.
(3) Trauma to the kidneys.
(4) Haematuria.

Urine protein levels are less than 0.07 mmol/1 per twenty-four hours.

Uraemia

This is the condition of raised blood urea. Normal blood urea is set at 1.0–6.0 mmol/1. Uraemia is caused by:

(1) Renal failure.
(2) Polycystic disease.
(3) Glomerulonephritis.
(4) Long-standing obstructions.
(5) Diabetes mellitus.

Haematuria

Blood in the urine has many causes, e.g.:

(1) Tumour.
(2) Calculi.
(3) Trauma.

Congenital abnormalities of the urinary tract

Fusion of kidneys ('Horseshoe kidney')

Horseshoe kidney (Figure 10.3) (Plate 10) results from anterior rotation of the kidneys. The kidneys fuse in the midline anterior to the aorta. Ninety per cent of all horseshoe kidneys fuse at the lower poles, which can cause obstruction and dilatation of the upper ureters. Other congenital abnormalities may be associated with the condition, although renal function is not generally impaired.

Ectopic kidney

During its development in the uterus, the kidney, or metanephros, migrates from the pelvis, where it is formed, into the abdomen. Failure of the kidney to rotate as it ascends results in a mal-rotated kidney. There is also

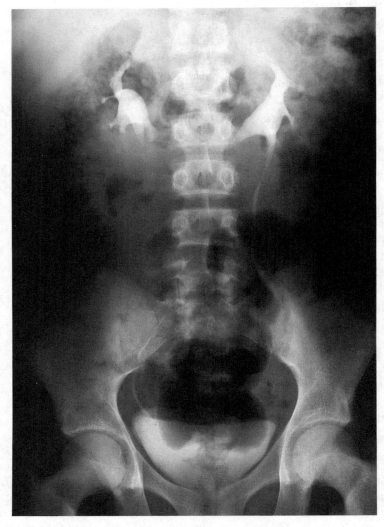

Plate 10   Horseshoe kidney connecting right and left kidneys

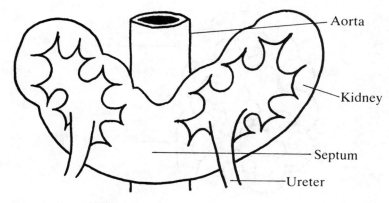

Figure 10.3   Horseshoe kidney

the possibility that the kidney may retain in the pelvis or migrate as far as the chest. This produces no interruption to normal renal function although the course of the ureters and blood vessels may appear very torturous. Ectopic kidneys may also be found in the lower part of the chest.

Agenesis/dysplasia

This is a complete failure in the development of the kidney or kidneys in utero. The ureter is also absent together with, in males, no seminal vesicles or vas deferens. Abnormal development of the kidney is referred to as dysplasia. Dysplastic kidneys still retain poorly defined areas of fetal kidney together with small cysts. Bilateral agenesis is incompatible with life. In unilateral agenesis there is usually compensatory hypertrophy of the other kidney.

Cysts

Simple

These are common and appear as variable sizes, usually in the cortex of the kidney, and in the majority of cases are detected incidentally. They are discrete fluid-filled cavities that have no connection with the renal pelvis. Gross enlargement may cause obstruction to the kidney. These cysts can be easily decompressed/aspirated under local anaesthetic through the skin under fluoroscopy or CT control.

Medullary sponge kidney

This congenital condition is usually first detected in children and adolescents, who most frequently present with recurrent urinary tract

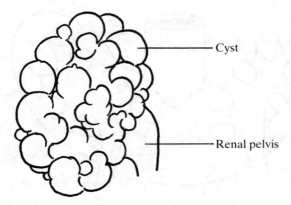

Figure 10.4   Polycystic disease

infections (UTI). The collecting tubules of the kidney become enlarged and dilated. Urine starts to pool in the tubules and calculi begin to form in the stagnant infected urine. Part or all of the kidney may be affected. In cross-section the medulla appears sponge-like, hence the name. Metabolic conditions associated with recurrent urinary calculi may also present in a similar way to medullary sponge kidney and must therefore be excluded.

The condition can be clearly diagnosed radiographically. Plain films of the renal area will show the presence of small calculi. Post-contrast radiographs of the kidney show the contrast medium pooling in the dilated tubules and filling defects in the collecting system caused by the calculi.

The patient experiences discomfort on passing small calculi. This may be relieved by performing a partial nephrectomy to remove areas of affected tissue.

Polycystic disease

This is an hereditary disease (Figure 10.4) that is inherited by both males and females. The condition is inherited as an autosomal dominant gene and is usually detected only in the fourth or fifth decade of life. As the disease develops the kidneys gradually become replaced by multiple cysts.

The patient usually presents with renal failure, haematuria, hypertension or they may present with an abdominal mass. On IVU the kidneys appear enlarged and the renal outline may be obscured by the presence of the cysts. Ultrasound is the examination usually preferred to diagnose the condition and differentiate between cysts and tumours.

The disease is associated with cysts in the lung, liver and pancreas and Berry cerebral aneurysms.

The disease is progressive and is controlled by giving the patient renal dialysis. Most patients also develop hypertension which must also be controlled. Surgery to the kidney is ineffective and is only carried out when the kidney becomes obstructed due to the presence of large cysts.

An infantile form of the disease is also known and is incompatible with life.

The development and course of polycystic disease is still little understood.

Duplex ureter

This is one of the commonest congenital malformations of the kidney (Figure 10.5). There is wide variation in the site and extent of division of the ureters.

As the kidney develops in utero the ureter grows out towards the developing kidney. The ureter branches to form the calyces as it nears the kidney. If the ureter branches very early on its path towards the kidney then duplex ureters are produced. If the ureter divides at a point closer to

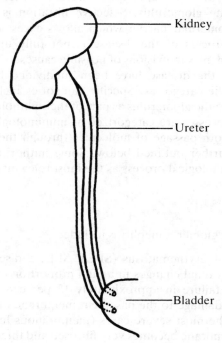

Figure 10.5   Duplex ureter

the kidney then the renal pelvis may appear bifid. If the ureters are joined at a point below the pelvis this may cause reflux of urine back up one element of the ureter.

In cases of complete duplex ureter the ureter draining the lower pole of the kidney has a normal insertion into the bladder. The upper pole ureter crosses the other ureter and usually has an ectopic insertion in the bladder, or, less frequently, in the urethra. The upper pole ureter can be obstructed by ureterocoele which can obstruct urine flow leading to dilatation and infection, hence damaging the kidney.

Glomerulonephritis

The kidney is divided into basic units called nephrons. These are responsible for the formation of urine formed by a process of selective filtration of the blood. The glomerulus, a network of capillaries, carries out filtration by retaining molecules with high molecular weights, e.g. blood cells and proteins, while allowing molecules with low molecular weights, e.g. waste products (urea, creatinine) to pass into the nephron.

Glomerulonephritis interrupts this filtration process by altering the permeability of the glomerulus. Selective filtration is impaired due to damage of the glomerular barrier which allows excess excretion of large molecules. The process of the disease is not fully understood as it is complex and has many subdivisions of possible causes.

The causes for the disease have been subdivided broadly into non-specific and specific categories. Specific categories include diseases that produce changes to the glomerulus as part of their pathological process.

Non-specific processes are categorized as immunological disorders that interrupt the smooth passage of molecules through the glomerulus. The two groups are further outlined below. Some authorities emphasize the non-specific immunological process as the most relevant cause of glomerular damage.

Specific

Specific causes for glomerulonephritis include:

(1) Systemic lupus erythematosus (SLE). SLE, a disease of connective tissues, causes renal changes in a high proportion of cases, and death due to renal failure in approximately 15 per cent of all cases. The extent of the damage to the basement membrane of the glomerulus is variable. In the most severe cases (membranous lupus nephritis) the basement membrane becomes very fibrosed and thickened.
(2) Diabetic renal disease (diabetic nephropathy). Patients with diabetes

mellitus develop premature generalized arteriosclerosis that thickens the basement membrane of the glomerulus. This restricts the permeability of the walls of the glomerulus and leads to glomerulonephritis.

Non-specific

Patients who suffer from a suppressed immunological system due to drugs or disease may also develop glomerulonephritis.

Any antigens present in the body are attacked and smothered by antibodies. The antibody-antigen complex is then passed to the kidneys by the reticulo-endothelial system. The complex then passes through the glomerulus into the urine. In patients with defective immune systems these immune complexes become lodged in the walls of the glomerulus and are not excreted. This prompts inflammatory changes in the basement membrane of the glomerulus. The wall becomes swollen and the normal cell structure breaks down. This again causes the retention of the waste products of metabolism and renal failure.

Hereditary causes: Alport's syndrome

This uncommon condition appears in boys and who usually show renal failure in childhood. The child presents with haematuria and proteinuria. The syndrome is also associated with deafness, bony abnormalities and neuropathy.

Course

Early changes due to glomerulonephritis are detected by the presence of albumen in the urine. As the disease progresses large amounts of protein appear in the urine together with some blood. Hypertension may also accompany the other symptoms. The disease may become particularly acute in patients with depressed immune systems.

If the disease is not checked then the glomeruli become scarred and replaced with fibrous tissue. Eventually the kidney appears shrunken and wasted and is described as 'end-stage kidney'. The kidney has grossly impaired or no function at this point and the patient requires renal dialysis or transplant to maintain life. Alport's syndrome often progresses to this point, the child requiring intensive dialysis.

An IVU carried out in the later stages of the disease will demonstrate a reduction in the renal size compared with earlier examinations, and poor renal function. However, the IVU is not carried out in isolation; the other clinical information and investigations are always considered together with the radiographic findings, e.g. ultrasound, CT, renography.

Urinary tract infection

Methods

There are three main routes through which the urinary tract becomes infected: (1) via the bloodstream, (2) through the outlet of the urinary system, and (3) through obstruction to the flow of urine.

Blood-borne

Blood-borne or haematogenous infection of the kidneys results in the formation of multiple small abscesses throughout the kidney. The spread of infection is in the form of small infected emboli that are carried in the blood from an area of infection remote from the kidney. In more advanced cases larger abscess cavities may form. Staphyloccus is the commonest organism underlying haematogenous urinary tract infection. Kidneys that have suffered damage or scarring from previous infections are more prone to subsequent infections.

From urinary outlet (ascending)

This type of infection results from bacteria ascending the urinary tract. Organisms may become introduced via the urethra and become lodged in the bladder. Urine in the bladder helps to culture the bacteria which may then spread throughout the urinary tract. Organisms commonly found in urine include: *Escherichia coli, Staphyloccocus pyogenes, Kleibsella, Streptoccocus faecalis.*

Obstruction to flow of urine

Organisms are present in the urine at all times. If the normal movement of urine is obstructed then the resulting stasis of urine will promote an infection.

Factors promoting infection

(1) Lowered resistance to infection. This is due to the presence of other disease or viruses that allow urinary tract infections to begin. Patients on immunosuppressants are also prone to infection.
(2) Presence of foreign bodies in the bladder or kidney, e.g. renal calculi.
(3) Fistulae formation from the bowel into the bladder due to Crohn's disease.
(4) Obstruction to the normal voiding of urine.

Results

Pyelonephritis

This is described as inflammation of the renal pelvis and renal parenchyma. The condition is divided into acute and chronic types.

Acute. The acute type commonly occurs:

(1) In childhood, when it is usually due to congenital abnormalities of the urinary tract.

(2) During pregnancy, due to obstruction of ureters by the uterus and physiological dilatation of the ureters and collecting systems.

(3) In the elderly, due to enlargement of the prostate in men and prolapse of the uterus in women. These cause obstruction to the bladder outflow and increased risk of infection.

Both haematogenous and ascending methods of infection are responsible for acute pyelonephritis, although haematogenous spread is thought to be the most common.

The kidney rapidly becomes damaged unless treatment is given. Small abscesses form and the kidney becomes damaged by the conversion of the renal parenchyma into fibrous tissue. The acute phase may progress to the chronic type of pyelonephritis.

IVU may show a swollen kidney with small elongated calyces that are distorted by the swollen renal parenchyma.

Chronic. As with other chronic infections, this results from multiple acute or low-grade infections. The kidneys appear shrunken and heavily scarred. Poor function is shown on IVU together with shrunken kidneys and loss of renal parenchyma. The changes are usually bilateral. A micturating cystogram may be carried out to demonstrate the reflux of urine. The renal changes are then complicated by hypertension and renal failure.

Interstitial. Interstitial nephritis also results from infections of the urinary tract. Reflux of infected urine into the kidney may form the focus of further infections. Interstitial nephritis is described by the area in which the infection becomes focused, e.g. cortical or medullary interstitial nephritis. Interstitial nephritis results from adverse drug reactions, e.g. as in a reaction to antibiotics. Drug abuse, particularly with analgesics, may also cause interstitial nephritis.

Complications

Papillary necrosis

Papillary necrosis indicates destruction of part or all of the papillae. This is as a result of an acute infection as in extensive interstitial infections. The renal papillae are sloughed off and are passed with the urine. This may occur in patients with diabetes. High analgesic intake, e.g. aspirin, may also cause papillary necrosis (analgesic abuse nephropathy).

The IVU may show filling defects within the calyces where the papillae have been destroyed. The necrotic papillae can also calcify prior to being sloughed off and pass down the ureter.

Calculus formation

Formation of renal calculi from whatever cause may follow urinary tract infection and stasis. The stone forms around bacteria within the urinary tract and, once formed, the urine is difficult to keep sterile.

Suppuration

Blood-borne infections may become complicated and deep-seated. This leads to formation of renal abscesses, and may be diagnosed with ultrasound. The kidney becomes very infected and requires intensive antibiotic therapy. The commonest causes for these abscesses are subacute bacterial endocarditis and osteomyelitis.

Granuloma

Granuloma develops following long-standing infections. The kidney initially suffers from interstitial infection which causes long-term inflammation and widespread formation of fibrous tissue. This may spread outside the boundary of the kidney and into other surrounding organs. The long-term presence of calculi, especially in diabetic patients, may also prompt the formation of granulomas.

Urinary tuberculosis

Urinary tuberculosis is caused by the blood-borne spread of *Mycobacterium tuberculosis,* usually from the chest. The absence of a visible focal lesion on a chest radiograph does not exclude tuberculosis in other systems.

The tubercle bacillus infects the cortex of the kidneys. Early stages of the infection may show as small irregularities of the renal papillae. The IVU may appear normal at this stage.

If untreated the infection progresses and causes abscess formation within the cortex. Formation of granulomas may also take place at later stages. These calcify and cause widespread damage to the kidney.

By this stage active tuberculous tissue has passed to the ureter and bladder. As the ureter becomes inflamed and scarred it becomes shorter and thicker. The bladder becomes thickened and smaller. The patient may experience haematuria and frequency as a result of the changes in the kidney and bladder.

Radiography of the urinary tract will show a variety of changes. Areas of calcification may be shown on plain radiographs. Contrast studies may show dilatation of the calices due to formation of fibrous tissue. The renal parenchyma becomes stretched preventing the flow of urine away from the calyces. This effect may also occur at the pelvi-ureteric junction and in the ureters causing obstruction and dilated ureters. The calyces may also have irregular shapes and become obliterated in cases of obstruction.

Involvement of the bladder will show as a poorly filled bladder with thickened walls. Multiple sites of involvement are commonly seen in tuberculosis.

The disease is detected by culturing tubercle bacillus from the urine. Treatment is given by antibiotic therapy and follow-up IVUs are carried out to monitor damage to the urinary tract. Occasionally surgical intervention is required to repair strictures caused by fibrous tissue formation.

Renal failure

Renal failure describes a complete loss of renal function and no production of urine. Renal failure is divided into acute and chronic types.

Acute

Acute renal failure is caused by:

(1) Severe trauma, e.g. following a major road accident whereby large amounts of blood and body fluids are lost leading to hypotension and poor circulation through the kidney.
(2) Surgery. Patients undergoing major heart surgery may go into renal failure. Myocardial ischaemia leading to hypotension may also cause renal failure.
(3) Severe burns, whereby large volumes of fluid are lost.
(4) Septicaemia following blood-borne infection, e.g. *Clostridium perfinges*.
(5) Retention of waste products due to inflammations and obstructions of the collecting systems. Large-scale cell damage as with papillary necrosis leads to blockage of the kidney and the build-up of toxic waste products.
(6) Intake of toxic substances, e.g. carbon tetrachloride.

Acute renal failure is divided into three phases: prodromal, anuria and recovery.

(1) Prodromal. Urine formation begins to drop. Small volumes of cloudy urine are formed in this phase.
(2) Anuria. This is the stage at which there is no urine production. The waste products of metabolism are retained in the body. Creatinine and other products build up at a rate determined by the underlying cause of the renal failure. In cases of severe infection, e.g. papillary necrosis, the rate is very high.
(3) Recovery. If the kidney has been severely damaged ('end-stage' kidney) then recovery is not possible and the patient must be given dialysis to survive. If the renal failure has been as a result of surgery then temporary dialysis may be given with an eventual return to normal function which is noted by a return to normal urine formation.

These three phases may take two to three weeks from start to finish. The end of the third phase comes with either recovery or loss of the kidney.

The patient in renal failure must be carefully managed. Fluid and food (protein) intake are carefully monitored to reduce the load placed on the kidneys. The amount of fluid given must equal the amount of fluid being lost through respiration and perspiration.

Chronic

Chronic renal failure may follow an episode of acute renal failure. Other renal disease, e.g. pyelonephritis, glomerulonephritis and congenital abnormalities such as polycystic disease also result in renal failure.

Long-term renal failure produces changes in the kidney and throughout the body. The bones commonly suffer osteomalacia leading to impaired uptake of calcium. Secondary hyperparathyroidism may also develop which causes loss of calcium from the bones (osteoporosis). Other symptoms of chronic renal failure include: hypertension, neuropathy, anaemia, general malaise, anorexia and weight loss.

Chronic renal failure may be controlled by limiting the protein intake and therefore the production of creatinine, etc. Renal failure usually results in the patient requiring some form of dialysis.

Renal dialysis

Two types of renal dialysis are used:

Peritoneal

A flexible catheter is inserted into the peritoneum of the patient (Figure

10.6) and dialysate fluid is run into the peritoneal space. This is then left *in situ* for 4–6 hours and then run out. This needs to be carried out four times per day. In the time that the fluid is in the peritoneum waste products are passed by osmosis into the fluid. Thus the peritoneum is being used as a semi-permeable membrane.

This is a widely used method of dialysis and allows the patient more freedom. The catheter is left *in situ* and the patient controls intake and release of fluid. This is known as continuous ambulatory peritoneal dialysis (CAPD) and can be carried out at the patient's place of work, etc.

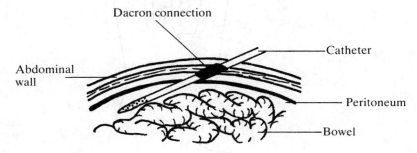

Figure 10.6   Peritoneal dialysis

Haemodialysis

In haemodialysis (Figure 10.7) blood flows from the patient's vessels through an artificial membrane. This allows diffusion of the waste products of metabolism into dialysate.

Blood at the patient's blood pressure travels from the body to the machine and back via a fistula. This is created by connecting a vein to an artery. The blood then travels in a complete integral loop. Fistula needles are inserted into the fistula at the time of dialysis to connect patient to the dialysis machine.

These Cimino fistulae are usually created in the radial artery. The veins become grossly enlarged due to the pressure exerted upon them by the arterial flow. The veins of the forearm become engorged by blood and may become blocked after continuous cannulation with the fistula needles.

If the dialysis is to be short term, as in post-operative patients, then a false arteriovenous shunt will be created. This Scribner shunt is composed of sialastic tubing and connects a vein to an artery under the skin surface. Needles are inserted into the catheter to complete the link to the dialysis machine. These are usually created in the leg, particularly with patients on ITU where access to the arms is often restricted.

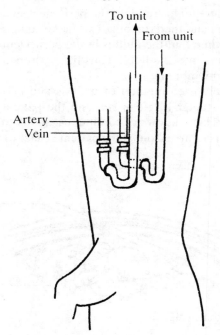

Figure 10.7   Creation of a fistula for renal dialysis

Patients undergo dialysis 2–3 times per week for 4–5 hours a session. The patient's diet must be restricted to reduce salt intake, and fluid intake is monitored to ensure that the amount taken in equals the amount lost.

Both methods carry the risk of infection, particularly in the case of CAPD, where poor hygiene may result in peritonitis. CAPD allows the patient to be more mobile and is by far the cheaper of the two methods.

Transplantation

Patients in renal failure may be sustained on dialysis for long periods. Renal transplant is a much more acceptable method of preserving life and alleviating the effects of renal failure. Kidneys for transplant are usually taken from patients who have been on respirators for extended periods and who have been declared dead. The kidneys are healthy because they have been perfused with fresh oxygenated blood. Kidneys from victims of road accidents tend to have suffered trauma through direct injuries and poor perfusion. Patients with a previous history of cancer are also excluded in order to rule out the possibility of tumour recurring. The ideal patient is one who has had a severe head injury or intracranial haemorrhage.

Transplanted kidneys are placed extraperitoneally in the iliac fossa. In children they may be placed more centrally. The renal vein is anastomosed to the external iliac vein and the renal artery to the internal or external iliac artery. The ureter is anastomosed to the bladder or a tunnel made into the wall of the bladder (Figure 10.8).

Rejection of the kidney by the body is the commonest reason for loss of function of the transplanted kidney. The body produces antigens that attempt to destroy the foreign tissue, as with any other antigen-antibody reaction.

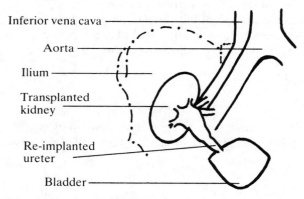

Inferior vena cava

Aorta

Ilium

Transplanted kidney

Re-implanted ureter

Bladder

Figure 10.8   Position of a transplanted kidney

Rejection takes place when an unrelated donor (allograft) is used. If a transplant is carried out between identical twins then no rejection takes place. Thus the implanted kidney is thought, by the host's antigens, to be its own tissue. Close tissue typing is carried out to prevent rejection as much as possible.

Immunosuppressive therapy and steriods are given to prevent rejection in the period after the transplant. The drug most commonly given is cyclosporin A. This is also given to patients undergoing other organ transplants. However, as immunosuppressants also suppress the bone marrow, their use must be carefully controlled. Large doses of steriod may also cause problems leading to ulceration of the upper gastrointestinal tract and Cushing's syndrome.

Mechanical problems leading to failure of the graft are now rare. The anastomosed renal artery may become stenosed. Reflux through the reinserted ureter may also occur.

The transplant kidney is monitored by carrying out isotope or ultrasound scans to check blood perfusion of the kidney, transplant arteriograms to check for mechanical damage, and needle biopsy to indicate any changes in the renal tissue.

The period at which rejection takes place is variable. Rejection may take place as soon as the surgeon allows the patient's blood to perfuse the transplanted kidney. This is called an hyperacute rejection and the kidney immediately takes on an unhealthy coloration. Urine formation commonly stops following transplant, but usually recovers. The rejected kidney fails due to infarction of the blood vessels within the kidney. A failed renal transplant must be removed to prevent widespread infection. The host's kidneys that are in renal failure are not removed.

If the first renal transplant fails then other transplants are attempted but prognosis with each subsequent attempt gets poorer. The patient is maintained on renal dialysis while another donor is located.

Renal calculi

Formation

All renal calculi require something around which they can form (a nidus). This may be provided by bacteria, fragments of dead tissue or foreign body.

Types

(1) Uric acid. Urates form stones in uric acid urine. Urates are soluble in alkaline urine. These occur more commonly in patients on chemotherapy.
(2) Amino acid (uncommon), e.g. cystine.
(3) Calcium carbonate/phosphate/oxalate. Most renal calculi are radio-opaque with the exception of pure uric acid calculi. Non-radio-opaque calculi may be seen as filling defeats on IVU. Ultrasound is very useful for detection of both radio-opaque and non-radio-opaque renal calculi.

Causes

(1) Hyperparathyroidism.
(a) Primary. In primary hyperparathyroidism increased excretion of parathyroid hormone causes mobilization of calcium from the skeleton leading to hypercalcaemia and hypercalcuria. Hypercalcuria causes formation of renal calculi. Increased release of calcium causes a fall in the level of phosphate in the plasma and osteoporosis.

(b) Secondary. Secondary hyperparathyroidism results from renal failure. Phosphate cannot be excreted in renal failure. This causes the amount of calcium in the blood to fall. The calcium is returned to the bones causing osteosclerosis or may deposit in the tissues or cause renal calculi. The fall in the level of calcium in the blood prompts the parathyroids to excrete more parathyroid hormone. The parathyroids undergo massive hypertrophy.

(2) Urinary infection. The presence of some bacteria in the urine aids calculi formation. The organism proteus mirabilis metabolizes urea into ammonia. This makes the urine alkaline and promotes the formation of calculi.

(3) Urinary stasis. Pooling of urine within the urinary tract due to obstruction of the kidney prompts the formation of stones. Lack of fluid movement simply gives the calculi time to form.

(4) pH of urine. Changes in the pH of the urine may prompt calculi formation.

(5) Chronic infections of the urinary tract.

(6) Papillary necrosis. Sloughing of the kidney's renal tubule by necrosis produces foci for the formation of calculi.

Complications of calculi formation

Calculi in the renal pelvis

Calculi in the renal pelvis cause obstruction to the flow of urine. The calculi often form in the calyces and become too large to pass into the ureters. The urine above the calculus may become infected and cause damage to the kidney. Obstruction to urine flow enhances growth of the stone. Presence of proteus mirabilis may cause the formation of large-scale stones that grow throughout the renal pelvis. These are called staghorn calculi which cause severe obstruction to urine flow and may lead to infection of the kidney and abscess formation.

Calculi in the ureter

Small calculi that pass from the calyces and then get lodged in the ureter (Figure 10.9) causing excruciating pain to the patient, 'renal colic'. The patient may vomit and the condition be taken as intestinal obstruction. The radiograph request form may show the confused request of 'Q. bowel obstruction, Q. calculus. Erect and supine abdo and CXR'.

Calculi that become stuck in the ureter cause proximal urinary stasis. Delayed IVU films show a distended renal pelvis with a dilated ureter above the level of the calculus.

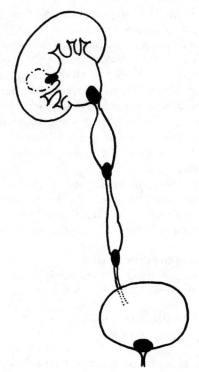

Figure 10.9   Common sites of renal calculi

Long-term obstruction will cause kidney damage, particularly if the patient's urine is infected. Obstruction can be relieved by nephrostomy under radiographic or ultrasound control. Calculi may be removed percutaneously through a nephrostomy. Lithotripsy and surgery are alternative methods for destruction and removal of calculi.

Calculi in the bladder

Some calculi may pass into the bladder but the majority of vesicle calculi arise in the bladder due to chronic bladder outflow obstruction. Small calculi are excreted via the urethra unless there is an outflow obstruction. The commonest cause of outflow obstruction in the adult male is prostatic hypertrophy. The calculus contained within the bladder grows in size as other mineral salts become deposited on its surface. This causes irritation to the wall of the bladder and may cause some haematuria. Bladder calculi are more common in men. Obstruction to the flow of urine commonly takes place at three points: (1) the pelvi-ureteric junction, (2) the vesico-ureteric junction and (3) the bladder outflow tract.

Treatment

In cases of renal colic the patient will be given pain relief. Radiographs are taken to assess the size of the calculus and cultures of the urine are taken to detect any infection. Large calculi may be removed by use of a variety of baskets and grasping instruments. These may be passed into the ureter via the bladder and the calculus removed.

Vascular conditions affecting the kidney

Aneurysms of the kidneys

Several types of aneurysm may be seen in relation to the blood supply to the kidney, e.g. saccular and fusiform.

Saccular aneurysms are prone to rupture or leak and must be repaired or resected and replaced by a dacron graft, or, in extreme cases, by removal of the aneurysm and kidney.

Arteriovenous malformations may develop in relation to carcinoma of the kidney. If associated with carcinoma the malformation is removed together with the kidney. Isolated arteriovenous malformations may be obliterated by carefully controlled embolisation under radiographic control.

Infarction

Infarction of the kidney may be focal, i.e. localized, or complete. The commonest cause of renal infarction is arterial. This frequently occurs through release of emboli from atheroma. Extensive acute infarctions are caused by either dissection of the atheromatous aorta or direct occlusion by atheroma. Venous occlusion usually results from the formation of large amounts of venous thrombosis, e.g. thrombosis of the IVC or iliac vessels by tumour or sepsis.

Trauma

Kidneys are usually protected from mild trauma by the lower ribs. Severe trauma to the kidney may result in a number of vascular changes including tearing of the renal arteries and veins, disruption of vessels within the kidney substance and tears through the renal parenchyma resulting in blood loss into the retroperitoneal part of the abdomen. Disruption of the renal vessels results in haemorrhage and renal failure. Trauma to the kidney is always treated as an emergency. The prime modalities for investigation of the kidney trauma are CT and ultrasound. Arteriography may also be used.

Hypertension

Renal artery stenosis

Renal artery stenosis may be caused by arteriosclerosis or be congenital due to fibromuscular dysplasia. This causes hypertension and damage to the kidney. If the disease becomes advanced, widespread damage to the kidney is caused by the effect of high blood pressure on the walls of the arteries.

Renal artery stenosis should be excluded in a relatively young hypertension patient. An IVU will show a delayed nephrogram and excretion on the affected side. Arteriography is carried out to show the position of the stenosis and the main treatment for this condition if angioplasty.

Renal failure

Hypertension can be caused by many diseases of the kidney, e.g. renal failure which causes disruption to the renin-angiotensin mechanism.

The juxtaglomerular apparatus lying around the afferent arteriole of the glomerulus secretes the enzyme renin in response to lowered blood pressure. Renin acts on angiotensinogen causing the further release of angiotensin I. Angiotensin I is then converted to angiotensin II. This increases the peripheral blood vessels and therefore causes an increase in blood pressure. Angiotensin II also causes the adrenal cortex to secret aldosterone. This causes the retention of sodium and the subsequent retention of water.

Usually, the release of renin and aldosterone balance each other by a feedback mechanism. Low sodium in the blood plasma will promote the release of renin. Damage to the adrenal glands, with a subsequent low release of aldosterone, will also result in increased secretion of renin. Disruption to the renal blood flow due to stenosis of the renal arteries may also affect the fine renin balance.

The levels of renin in the blood plasma may be measured under radiographic control. A catheter is positioned in the abdominal aorta and blood samples are taken above, below and at the level of the renal arteries and veins. Angiograms may then be carried out to detect any narrowing in the diameter of the renal artery.

Conn's syndrome (rare cause of hypertension)

Conn's disease, or primary hyperaldosteronism, is caused by single or multiple adenomas of the zona glomerulosa in the adrenal glands. The tumours are rarely malignant. The adenoma secretes aldosterone. This results in the retention of sodium which leads to hypertension.

Spironolactone may be given which counteracts the effects of aldosterone. However this drug has unpleasant side-effects and surgery to the adrenals is usually carried out. The adrenal adenoma must be accurately located, e.g. by CT scanning. If an adenoma is found within the gland then the whole gland is removed.

Tumours of the kidney

Malignant tumours of the renal parenchyma

Adenocarcinoma (Grawitz tumour)

This is a malignant renal tumour occurring mainly at 50–60 years of age. It is very rare before puberty. Occurrence is twice as common in men as in women.

It is thought that the tumours arise from pre-existing cortical adenomas. The tumours present as large rounded masses that cause cystic and necrotic areas. The tumours are often encapsulated and are yellow due to the breakdown of lipids. They may be graded into three groups of varying malignancy. These are decided by the degree of tissue differentiation within the tumour:

Grade I has the best prognosis with well-differentiated cells.

Grade II, moderately well-differentiated cells.

Grade III. Poor prognosis with poor differentiation of cells within the tumour.

The tumour spreads by direct invasion throughout the renal substance. Spread is also into the renal vein, promoting the spread of secondaries to the lungs and bones. Lymphatic spread also takes place.

The patient usually presents with haematuria and pain. They may also be aware of the mass and suffer from weight loss.

Invasion of the renal vein giving rise to haematuria usually indicates a later stage of the disease and is associated with a poor prognosis. Grading of the tumour is important in determining the prognosis. Twenty per cent of patients with a Grade I-type tumour and a complete nephrectomy have a survival period of ten years.

The tumour is very vascular and demonstrated angiographically.

Ultrasound and/or CT are the modality of choice to diagnose and demonstrate the extent of the tumour to distinguish the mass from renal cysts.

Wilm's tumour (primitive cell tumour)

This forms about 10 per cent of all malignant renal tumours. The majority of Wilm's tumours occur before the age of six or seven years. Ten per cent of the tumours are bilateral. It has an equal distribution between males and females.

The tumour usually presents as a large abdominal mass in a child. The tumour is composed of embryonic tissue which includes muscle fibres, bone and connective tissues. The tumour grows rapidly as an isolated mass. The tumour rarely invades the renal pelvis.

Spread of the tumour is by direct invasion of surrounding tissues. Lymphatic and secondary spread into the bones is common. Haematuria, weight loss and other features such as blood disorders usually occur at a late stage in the disease.

The child is treated by radical nephrectomy of the affected kidney. In the case of bilateral Wilm's careful arteriography is carried out to plan partial nephrectomies. Exploration of other abdominal organs is carried out to exclude metastatic spread of the tumour. Radiotherapy is given to the kidney bed and a chemotherapy drug regime is set up.

Secondary tumours of the renal parenchyma

Secondary involvement of the kidneys may be seen but they are a comparatively unusual site for metastatic disease, despite the one-fifth of the total blood volume perfusing the kidneys.

Tumours of the renal pelvis and ureter

These rare tumours are more frequently seen in the elderly. They are usually malignant and classification of the malignancy of the tumour is made as in bladder tumours (see p. 231). The tumour arises in the renal pelvis and spreads to involve the ureter. There are often multiple lesions but bilateral incidence of tumours in the renal pelvis is uncommon. Two types of tumour occur in the renal pelvis:

(1) Transitional (urothelial) cell type.
(2) Squamous cell type. These are associated with long-standing calculi causing dysplasia which leads to malignant change of the epithelium in the renal pelvis. They are very malignant and highly invasive.

The tumours spread via the lymphatics, the bloodstream, commonly to the lungs, and by direct spread to the bladder and ureter. Haematuria and obstruction to the kidney are common presentations of the tumour.

Tumours of the adrenal gland

Phaeochromocytoma

This is a tumour of the adrenal medulla which secretes adrenaline and noradrenaline. They act as neurotransmitters. Increased concentration of these catecholamines causes persistent and paroxysmal hypertension.

The presence of increased levels of noradrenaline and adrenaline may be measured by analysis of the blood plasma or urine. The urine contains the breakdown products of the catecholamines. One product is called vannilyl-mandelic acid (VMA). Measuring the level of this chemical indicates the level of catecholamines in the blood.

Phaeochromocytomas are very vascular and are detected by high dose IVU with tomography and by arteriography.

Surgical removal is usually carried out and the patient is prepared for surgery by giving drugs that block the effects of the adrenaline and noradrenaline. Being vascular tumours they are usually embolised by radiologists prior to surgery.

Phaeochromocytomas may also develop outside the adrenal gland in other areas of the abdomen.

THE BLADDER

The bladder wall is composed of:

(1) An inner transitional epithelium.
(2) The tunica propria which is a layer of connective tissue.
(3) A muscle layer. The smooth muscle fibres making up the bladder wall form a dense network around the ureteric openings and the internal urethal meatus. These areas act as sphincters controlling entrance and exit of fluids.
(4) Serosa. An outer covering of epithelium.

Figure 10.10 shows the basic structure of the bladder.

Inflammations

Acute cystitis

This is a common condition, particularly in women. The bladder becomes inflamed due mainly to *Escherichia coli* and *Streptococcus faecalis*. These

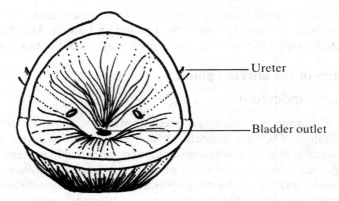

Figure 10.10　Structure of the bladder

bacteria are found in the bowel and may invade the female urethra. Other causes of inflammation are chemicals and non-bacterial organisms. Infection may also develop in the bladder by bacteria descending the ureter or being transported by the lymphatics.

The urine becomes quickly colonized by the micro-organisms and appears cloudy and smells of ammonia. The patient also feels the urge to micturate at frequent intervals. The mucosa becomes inflamed and painful and the patient has dysuria.

The condition is treated with antibiotics and usually resolves. If the cystitis is not effectively treated then the condition will become chronic. If untreated the bladder may become shrunken and contracted.

Cystitis in men usually underlies something more serious, e.g. a calculus in the bladder or kidney.

Other types of cystitis

Interstitial (Hunner's ulcer)

The mechanism of the formation of Hunner's ulcer is not fully understood. An area of the bladder undergoes changes that result in the muscle layer of the bladder becoming heavily fibrosed. This results in a grossly contracted bladder with a very low capacity. The bladder may require partial resection and replacement with a portion of caecum.

Encrusted

In this condition the walls of the bladder become coated with precipitated white urinary salts. This is caused by the presence of urea-splitting organisms such as proteus mirabilis. This may cause loss of volume and a fibrotic bladder. Extensive use of antibiotics is made to control the organism.

Disturbances to micturition

Micturition

Pressure receptors in the wall of the bladder pass afferent impulses to the sacral (S2–S3) segments of the spinal cord. These impulses carry information about the amount of urine contained within the bladder. Efferent impulses are passed back that stimulate the detrusor muscle to contract and cause voiding of the bladder. This mechanism is usually under the control of the higher centres. Hence the patient has control over the amount of urine contained in the bladder prior to voiding. In micturition the patient must allow relaxation of the external sphincter. There are a number of conditions in which there is a disruption to this pathway of control of micturition.

Urodynamics

This is the study of the pressures in the bladder and contraction of the detrusor muscle under radiographic control. A catheter attached to a transducer is placed in the bladder to measure the intravesical pressure. A second catheter and pressure line is inserted into the rectum, measuring intra-abdominal pressure. An electronic system is used that subtracts the intra-abdominal pressure from the intravesical pressure to give the true pressure acting on the detrusor muscle. The rectal pressure, intravesical pressure and the subtracted pressure are recorded on a paper trace.

The bladder is filled with saline containing a contrast medium that allows the filling to be observed under radiographic control. The filling and emptying are recorded on video.

Disorders of micturition

Over-stimulation

The presence of a calculi or infection will cause irritation of the mucosa in the bladder and lead to over-stimulation of the detrusor, and so to frequent micturition, when small amounts of urine are voided.

Paraplegia

If the spinal cord is severed above the level of S2 and S3 segments of the spinal cord then the bladder mechanisms become isolated from the higher centres. The patient then has no control over voiding. The sphincters controlling release of the urine do not work in co-ordination with the detrusor muscle. The detrusor pushes against the unrelaxed sphincters which leads to hypertrophy of the detrusor. The bladder becomes floppy and characteristically pear-shaped and retains urine which leads to infections.

Urodynamic studies of the paraplegic bladder show uncontrolled swings in detrusor pressure as the bladder begins to fill. The pressure rises to very high levels and then drops at irregular intervals.

Surgery to the pelvis to remove extensive tumour growth may result in damage to the parasympathetic nerves carrying impulses to the spinal cord from the bladder. This results in a large over-distended bladder with the external sphincter acting as an outflow obstruction to the flow of urine.

Prolapsed bladder

Degrees of vesical neck prolapse are encountered in women who have given birth per vagina. This is due to laxity of the pelvic muscles, specifically the levatore ani muscle, which leads to downwards herniation of the bladder neck and sphincter. The subsequent loss of control over the external sphincter results in voiding of urine as a result of coughing, laughing, etc. This is called stress incontinence as opposed to urge incontinence which develops as a result of bladder infections. Stress incontinence may be surgically or medically corrected.

Bladder outflow obstruction

This is usually due to urethral strictures or enlarged prostate. The obstruction results in a grossly hypertrophied bladder (Figure 10.11). The bladder wall is thickened and the patient suffers from frequency and urgency of micturition.

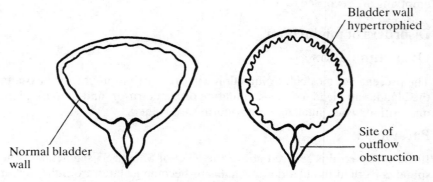

Figure 10.11   Obstruction of the bladder neck causes changes to the bladder wall

Cancer of the bladder

Three per cent of all malignant tumours are accounted for by bladder tumours. These commonly occur in the sixth and seventh decades and are more common in men.

Certain factors have been shown to favour the production of bladder cancers. People working with dyes, particularly analine-type dyes have been shown to have a higher incidence of bladder tumours. Smoking is also indicated as a significant factor in bladder tumours.

Types

The tumours may occur as single or multiple lesions and are commonly locally malignant. Most tumours are of the papillary cell type arising from the surface epithelium and growing into the lumen of the bladder. Ulcerative and nodular forms of tumour also occur. These also arise from the surface epithelium and invade the bladder wall. They carry a poorer prognosis than the papillary type. Squamous cell carcinomas may also occur and are usually associated with vesicle calculi.

Spread

Spread is by direct invasion of surrounding tissues and by infiltration to the draining lymph nodes, e.g. to the iliac groups of nodes and then on to the para-aortic nodes. Metastases can occur in the bones, liver and lungs. The patient presents with haematuria and dysuria.

Staging

The tumours are staged by the degree of infiltration of the bladder wall. T indicates a superficial tumour. T1 is a tumour that has infiltrated the submucosa. T2 is superficial involvement and T3 deep muscle involvement. T4 tumours are neoplasms that have invaded adjacent organs (UICC classification).

Treatment/management

The majority of bladder tumours are managed by cystoscopy and diotherapy. T3 and T4 tumours require more radical surgery with cystectomy and removal of adjacent structures. An ileal loop is formed and ureters implanted into it. This is periodically and passively compressed by the patient to void urine through an ileostomy. The surgery is supported by treatment with radiotherapy. The five-year survival rate for patients with advanced cancers following radical surgery is 20–30 per cent.

THE REPRODUCTIVE SYSTEM

The prostate gland

The prostate gland (Figure 10.12) lies at the base of the bladder. It surrounds the upper part of the urethra and the posterior aspect is closely aligned to the rectum. The bulk of the gland is composed of fibromuscular and glandular tissues.

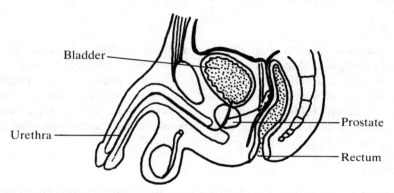

Bladder

Urethra

Prostate

Rectum

Figure 10.12   Sagittal section of the male pelvis

Benign enlargement

Benign enlargement of the prostate gland is very common in men over the age of forty. This is due to hyperplasia of the gland. The muscle and glandular tissues within the gland undergo hypertrophy which results in the prostate gland obstructing the outlet of the bladder. This insidious bladder obstruction causes hypertrophy and increased trabeculation of the bladder wall as the bladder attempts to empty the urine. The patient experiences frequency of micturition as there is a varying amount of urine remaining after micturition.

Hypertrophy of the bladder wall produces two effects on the ureters:

(1) The lower end of the ureters becomes narrowed. This can cause partial obstruction to the flow of urine into the bladder which increases the risk of infection.
(2) The vesico-ureteric valve at the lower end of the ureter can become incompetent which leads to reflux of the urine back into the calyces. This carries the risk of glomerulonephritis.

Eventually the detrusor muscle loses the ability to maintain the pressure against the obstruction and becomes flaccid and lacking in tone. The failure of the detrusor muscle means that the patient cannot micturate. This may occur quite suddenly. The bladder becomes distended and the patient experiences great discomfort. This necessitates catheterization of the bladder and urgent surgery to the prostate to relieve the obstruction.

Appearances

Ultrasound is the first examination of choice to check the state of kidneys, collecting systems, bladder and prostate. An IVU may be carried out to show the anatomy of the bladder and kidneys in the patient with suspected prostate problems. The examination will show an hypertrophied, thick-walled bladder and a large prostate at its base with some residual urine following micturition.

Malignant tumours

Cancer of the prostate is very common in males in their seventh and eighth decades. The symptoms are very similar to those found with benign hyperplasia of the prostate. The patient suffers from retention of urine. Biopsy of the gland reveals the extent of the tumour.

Staging

Prostate tumours are classed as adenocarcinomas. The extent of the tumour is summarized into four main groups. Other subdivisions are also used:

T1 is a tumour confined to the prostate that is surrounded by normal tissue.
T2 is a tumour confined to the prostate gland.
T3 indicates a tumour that has extended beyond the gland capsule with or without involvement of the lacteral sulci and/or the seminal vesicles.
T4 is either a fixed tumour or a tumour invading adjacent structures (TNM classification).

The extent of the tumour is gauged by carrying out bone scans, CT scans and lymphography. The tumour metastasises via the bloodstream and lymphatics mainly to the bones which are characteristically sclerotic.

Treatment

Complete or partial removal of the prostate is generally necessary. This depends on the extent of the disease. This will usually be complemented by radiotherapy. It has also been found that treatment with oestrogen and other synthetic oestrogens, e.g. trichloroansene (TACE), has helped control the growth of the tumour as the tumour can be testosterone stimulated.

The removal of both testes (bilateral orchidectomy) has also been shown to control the spread of the tumour. Chemotherapy is not found to be very successful for prostatic cancers.

The urethra

In males, the urethra forms the outflow pathway for both urine and seminal fluid. The male urethra is approximately 20 cm long, extending from the tip of the penis to the base of the bladder. The first portion runs through the prostate.

The female urethra follows a much less torturous course than the male urethra. The opening of the female urethra is in close proximity to the vagina and rectum.

Stricture of the urethra

This is usually due to infections, especially venereal, or trauma to the urethra. Fibrous tissue forms in the urethra following infection which results in narrowing of the bore of the urethra.

The stricture results in the retention of urine in the bladder. This promotes the formation of urinary tract infections. Dilation of the urethra beyond the point of the stricture may promote formation of infections and calculi. The stricture may be demonstrated radiographically by introducing contrast medium into the urethra and carefully recording the point of the stricture. The stricture is relieved under general anaesthetic by using dilators or bougies to open out the narrowing.

Inflammations

Non-specific urethritis

This describes a group of infections, usually transmitted after sexual intercourse that lead to dysuria, frequency of micturition and a discharge per urethrum.

Gonococcal urethritis

This may be caused by *Neissaria gonorrhoeae* and is contracted during sexual intercourse, usually with an infected partner. The organism produces an acute urethritis that may cause local lymph node involvement together with a purulent exudate and dysuria. The pus smears show dense populations of gonococci.

The testes

These lie within the scrotum and are composed of three basic tissue layers:

(1) The tunica vaginalis. This is composed of two layers separated by a film of serous fluid.
(2) The tunica albuginea. This is the middle layer and is composed of fibrous tissue.
(3) The tunica vasculosa. This inner layer is composed of areolar tissue and contains a plexus of blood vessels.

Hydrocoele

This is a common condition caused by an accumulation of fluid in the tunica vaginalis (Figure 10.13). The cause is usually idiopathic, but may be associated with trauma, or it may be congenital or due to the presence of inflammations or neoplasms. Congenital hydrocoeles may also be associated with inguinal hernia or undescended testes. Hydrocoeles are generally drained. The aspirated fluid is rich in proteins. Other types of collections within the tunica vaginalis include: haematocoele and spermatocoele. These are named by their content.

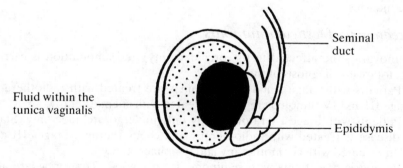

Seminal duct

Fluid within the tunica vaginalis

Epididymis

Figure 10.13   A hydrocoele

Tumours

Seminomas

Seminomas account for 35–40 per cent of all testicular tumours. In all classifications seminomas are taken to be of germ cell origin and occur in children and adults. The tumour presents as a painless swelling that may be bilateral. The swelling is usually restricted to the seminiferous epithelium but may spread to the epididymis by direct invasion. The tumour may also spread to the local lymph nodes and spread to the para-aortic nodes.

Secondary spread via the blood commonly occurs to the lung, liver, brain and bones.

Teratoma

Approximately 30 per cent of all testicular tumours are of this type. Teratomas do not have the clear-cut histology of the seminoma. Teratomas are divided into four main groups:

(1) Differentiated teratoma. This contains clearly differentiated tissue.
(2) Malignant teratoma intermediate. This contains both differentiated and malignant cells.
(3) Malignant teratoma. This shows an absence of differentiated tissue and is composed of purely cancerous tissue.
(4) Malignant teratoma trophoblastic. This final type is composed of cancer tissue which must be of a specific tumour type, e.g. papillary.

Teratoma spreads via the bloodstream, commonly to the lungs and liver.

Staging

Staging is carried out by CT, lymphography and lung tomography to detect secondaries.

Treatment of testicular tumours

Removal of the affected testis (orchidectomy) and amputation is carried out following diagnosis of the tumour.

Patients with Stage I and II seminomas are treated with radiotherapy. Stage III and IV tumours are further treated with chemotherapy.

Patients with Stage I teratomas may only undergo orchidectomy. Stage II disease is treated with radiotherapy and chemotherapy. Stages III and IV are treated with chemotherapy and lymphadectomy.

Prognosis of patients with seminoma is very good. Teratomas are also successfully treated, although advanced malignant teratomas have a poor prognosis.

The uterus

The uterus is subdivided into the body and the cervix. The cervix comprises the lower part of the uterus and is approximately 2.5 cm in length (Figure 10.4). The wall of the uterus is composed of three coats:

(1) An outer peritoneal coat.
(2) A middle muscular coat (myometrium).

(3) An inner mucous coat (endometrium) which is continuous with the uterine tubes above and the vagina below.

Endometrial polyps

These may be multiple or single and have a variable composition. Single polyps are usually cystic and surrounded by unaffected secretory tissue. Multiple polyps may disrupt function over wider areas.

Uterine fibroids (leiomyomas)

These are benign tumours of the myometrium that are composed of smooth muscle and fibrous tissue. They arise from the uterine muscle and their continued growth depends upon oestrogens. Fibroids are a very common form of tumour and start to form in very young females. They usually cause no symptoms and atrophy after the menopause. However they are prone to change and may undergo ossification and fatty degeneration.

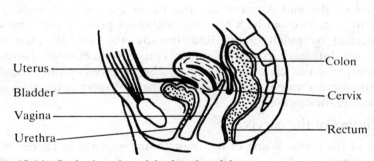

Figure 10.14   Sagittal section of the female pelvis

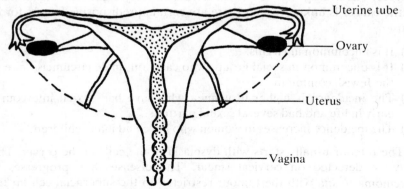

Figure 10.15   Position of the ovaries

Malignant tumours of the endometrium

Endometrial malignant tumours can occur from any part of the endometrial epithelium. The tumour initially grows into the uterine cavity, but later spreads into the underlying muscles. The vagina and adjacent organs may also become involved. Endometrial polyps are not usually thought of as being precursors of malignancy.

The patient presents with vaginal discharge and bleeding. Ultrasound may show an enlarged uterus and differentiation between muscle and uterine cavity. Only direct biopsy gives an accurate diagnosis.

Tumours of the endometrium are regarded as adenocarcinomas. Sarcomas of the uterus are rare, and are thought to arise from fibroids.

Spread of the uterine tumour is very slow as the wall of the uterus provides an efficient barrier to the spread of disease. The disease usually spreads by involvement of the external iliac and hypogastric nodes.

Treatment

Tumours of the endometrium are treated in a variety of ways. Hysterectomy is carried out with bilateral salpingo-oophorectomy. This may be preceded by radiotherapy. Radiotherapy may also be used post-operatively. Intracavitary radium implants may also be inserted. Hormone treatment, to arrest cancer growth, may also be given. With T1 and T2 types the survival rate is very good. The length of survival depends upon the extent of the disease.

Carcinoma of the cervix

Cancer of the cervix is one of the most common causes of cancer in the female population. It accounts for 4 per cent of all deaths from malignant disease. The average age of women affected is forty-eight. The actual cause of the cancer is unknown, but there are certain predisposing factors for its cause:

(1) It is uncommon in virgins.
(2) It is uncommon in social groups who carry out male circumcision, e.g. the Jewish community.
(3) The incidence is higher in women who have had sexual intercourse early in life and had several sexual partners.
(4) The incidence increases in women who have had many children.

The tumour usually starts with dysplasia of the cells in the cervix. This may be detected on cervical smear. The disease then progresses to carcinoma *in situ* with the tumour restricted to the superficial cell layers. The tumour then begins to invade the underlying tissues.

More than 95 per cent of all uterine cancers are squamous cell carcinomas.

Staging

Stage 0. Carcinoma *in situ.*
Stage 1. Confined to cervix.
Stage 1a. Micro-invasive.
Stage 1b. Invasive.
Stage II. Direct spread to other extra-cervical tissue, but not to lower third of vagina.
Stage III. Involvement of pelvic wall and lower third of vagina.
Stage IVa. Extension to the bladder, rectum and beyond the true pelvis.
Stage IVb. Distant organs. (FIGO classification.)

Diagnosis

Detection of cervical cancer is conducted through many tests, mainly cervical smears and biopsy.

Treatment

Treatment of cervical cancer depends upon the stage of the disease. Early stages may require removal of part of the cervix. In more advanced cases the cancer is treated by hysterectomy and intracavity irradiation. Chemotherapy is also used, e.g. cis-platinum. Prognosis depends upon the extent of the disease.

The ovaries

These lie on either side of the uterus (Figure 10.15). Each is composed of two layers:

(1) The medulla. This is a layer of connective tissue.
(2) The cortex. This contains a complex layer of germinal epithelium that gives rise to the ovum.

Cancer

There are many types of ovarian carcinoma. They account for about 3 per cent of all deaths due to malignancies. The tumours are grouped into a number of classes, examples of which are:

(1) Epithelial tumours. These are the commonest of the ovarian tumours and are further subdivided into other histological groups, e.g. serous, mucinous, endometroid and clear cell.
(2) Sex cord stromal tumours. These are thought to be derived from the

gonadal mesenchyme which has the potential to differentiate into male or female gonads.

(3) Germ-cell tumours. These arise from the germinal cells. This group includes teratomas.

(4) Other types of tumour arising from the ovary.

Staging of ovarian tumours

Stage I. Limited to ovaries.
Stage II. Showing pelvic extension.
Stage III. Extension to bowel.
Stage IV. Distant organs. (FIGO classification.)

Treatment

Hysterectomy with bilateral salpingo-oophrectomy is the prime treatment of choice. Chemotherapy is used in combination with the surgery.

Abnormalities of sexual development

Klinefelter's syndrome (XXY)

The presence of the extra Y chromosome leads to development of male characteristics with some testicular development.

Turner's syndrome (XO)

This occurs in women. The lack of a second X chromosome leads to failure of the formation of gonads. This produces a sterile female with abnormalities throughout the body including the cardiovascular system. It is treated with replacement hormone therapy.

11
BONE AND JOINT DISEASE

THE BONES

Structure

Bone is a connective tissue and is composed from a matrix of water, collagen and mineral salts. The major mineral in bone is calcium in the form of calcium hydroxyapatite. Cross-section of a living bone shows three layers (Figure 11.1):

(1) The periosteum.
(2) The cortex.
(3) The medulla.

The periosteum

The bone is covered by an outer layer of tissue called the periosteum. This is composed of an outer fibrous layer and an inner osteogenic layer. In young immature bones the periosteum is highly vascular and very active. Osteoblasts lying within the periosteum produce new bone onto the bony surface.

The periosteum ensheathes any tendons, nerves or blood vessels attached to the bone and is only usually absent at the articular surfaces of the bone. The periosteum communicates with the underlying bone via blood vessels running down through bony cortex. Loss of the periosteum results in death of the bone.

The Cortex

The cortex is composed of compact bone. This consists of units called

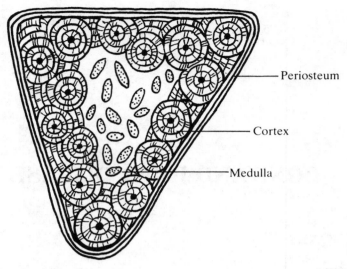

Figure 11.1   Structure of bone

Haversian systems or secondary osteons. These are roughly cylindrical and have at their centre an Haversian canal. This has a number of vessels running through it that include a nerve fibre, capillary vessel, lymph vessel and a vein.

The Haversian canals are surrounded by concentric rings of lamellar bone. Lying between these concentric lamellae are small spaces called lacunae that link together via fine channels called canaliculi. The lacunae contain the bone cells or osteocytes and the canaliculi provide canals for the connections between the osteocytes.

The surface of the compact bone becomes marked with trabecular lines that follow the lines of stress applied to the bone.

The medulla

The medullary cavity, lying at the centre of the bone, is composed of a much more porous type of bone called cancellous or spongy bone. Cancellous bone forms a loose trabecular pattern within which lies the bone marrow.

Bone marrow occurs as red and yellow marrow. At birth the marrow in the skeleton is red. This is gradually replaced by yellow marrow until in the adult it only remains in the sternum, ribs, ileac and long bones. Red marrow is responsible for the production of red blood cells and is supplied by the nutrient artery which supplies and collects blood from the bone.

The ratio of compact bone to cancellous bone varies according to the stresses applied to the bone. Bones that bear weight show a higher proportion of compact bone.

Loss of bone density (osteopenia)

Osteopenia on radiographs is seen as a rarefaction of the bone. This is often difficult to detect radiographically especially in the early stages. Radiographs are sometimes taken of dry bones with a known standard of calcium content to compare with bones that are thought to be osteoporotic. Decreased bone density can be due to osteoporosis, rickets or osteomalacia, or other endocrine disorders. Each of the main disease processes are outlined below.

Osteoporosis

Osteoporosis is a condition of bone atrophy resulting in a reduction in the volume of bone matrix without any change in the composition of the remaining bone matrix. Osteoporosis may be detected by measuring the levels of calcium and phosphatase in the blood and urine. Radioisotope bone scans may also be used because they are useful indicators of bone metabolism.

In osteoporosis the normal trabecular pattern of the bone is disrupted. The trabeculae become more apparent when seen in the spine and the edges of the vertebral bodies become well defined. This leaves the bones brittle and weakened and therefore liable to break easily. Fractures of the wrist and neck of femur are common and occur with the minimum amount of force. Crush fractures of the vertebral bodies may also occur leading to the characteristics kyphosis found in the elderly.

The cause of the loss of bone matrix may be due to either loss of osteoblast activity and the subsequent failure of the bone tissue to lay down new bone, or increased osteoclast activity. Osteoporosis may be idiopathic, or associated with immobilization or disease.

Causes

Idiopathic

This is the commonest type of osteoporosis. Idiopathic osteoporosis is often subdivided according to age, e.g. juvenile (very uncommon), post-menopausal and senile (the commonest).

In the elderly it is thought to be due to the atrophy associated with ageing. Osteoblast activity slows and the matrix becomes rarified.

Fractures of the wrist and neck of femur are common in the elderly and occur with the minimum amount of force. Crush fractures of the spine can also occur, giving the characteristic kyphoses and scolioses of elderly patients.

Post-menopausal osteoporosis in women is thought to be due to lack of oestrogen in the bloodstream. The oestrogen seems to maintain the normal bone structure. The increased incidence of fractures in elderly women is thought to be due to low blood oestrogen levels. Thus post-menopausal treatment with oestrogen may be given to women to prevent osteoporosis.

Prolonged immobilization

Prolonged immobilization, e.g. due to bed rest, produces an increase in the excretion of calcium (hypercalcuria). In some cases the amount of calcium excreted may cause renal calculi formation. The resulting osteoporosis may cause severe bone weakness. A similar effect may be seen in a limb immobilized for long periods in a plaster cast.

Scurvy (rare cause of osteoporosis)

Vitamin C (ascorbic acid) is essential in the formation of collagen fibres. Collagen comprises almost 90 per cent of the bone matrix. Therefore lack of vitamin C results in rarefaction of the bones and osteoporosis. In adults this leads to a general rarefaction of bone. In children the disease is more complex and results in impaired bone formation and fracture of the epiphysis.

Hyperthyroidism

Thyrotoxicosis produces mild osteoporosis due to increased osteoclast activity, which cannot be detected on conventional radiographs.

Osteogenesis imperfecta (fragilitas ossium)

This congenital disease may appear at birth or during infancy. (It rarely appears during adolescence.) It is characterized by a defect in bone formation causing the bones to be osteoporotic and very fragile. The bones bend and fracture very easily giving rise to a very deformed skeleton. Osteogenesis imperfecta is a genetically linked disease.

Cushing's syndrome

Over-production or ingestion of glucocorticoids or adenocorticotrophic hormone (ACTH) produces osteoporosis. This is thought to be due to the suppression of normal osteoblast activity.

Loss of bone minerals

This is the second group of diseases that produce osteopenia. In osteoporosis, the composition of the remaining bone matrix was unaffected. In diseases such as vitamin D deficiency, bone rarefaction takes place due to a decrease in the bone mineral content. In bone demineralization the blood shows a decreased level of calcium. Loss of bone mineral may be associated with rickets and hyperparathyroidism.

Rickets (vitamin D deficiency)

Vitamin D is responsible for the absorption of calcium from the ileum and the deposition of calcium salts in the bone. Vitamin D is also synthesized in the skin in small amounts. Rickets (Figure 11.2) is uncommon in Great Britain but still occurs in some immigrant communities and some underdeveloped countries. Vitamin D deficiency produces changes in the skeleton where maximum growth is taking place, at the epiphyseal regions, i.e. the points where calcium is being deposited. The growth plate lying between the metaphysis and epiphysis from which calcification takes place becomes irregularly calcified and ragged.

The bones may become weakened and may shorten or bend. Young bones affected by rickets are prone to greenstick fractures.

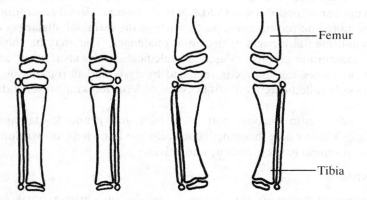

Figure 11.2   Rickets: unaffected legs (left) and affected legs (right)

Osteomalacia

Osteomalacia is an adult form of rickets. Normal adult bone is constantly being renewed by osteoclast activity. The bone is replaced by osteoid, an intermediate tissue that promptly calcifies to form new bone. If the osteoid fails to calcify then the whole bone remains in the osteoid form. The bone appears osteoporotic with a thinning and loss of trabeculae and bone cortex. The mineral content of the bone is again very low and this leads to the signs found in rickets, especially deformities of the limbs. Fractures of the bones may also occur. These are usually small and marked by areas of sclerosis and ossified callus, so-called 'looser zones'.

Osteomalacia occurs as a result of vitamin D deficiency and reduced calcium intake. This may be as a result of malabsorption or inadequate diet.

Hyperparathyroidism

Parathyroid hormone promotes the resorption and remodelling of bone by stimulating the action of osteoclasts. The hormone also stimulates increased excretion of calcium by the kidneys. In hyperparathyroidism, the level of parathyroid hormone increases and accelerates the action it has on bone tissue. The disease is divided into primary and secondary forms.

Primary

Primary hyperparathyroidism is due to tumours or increased activity of the parathyroid glands over-secreting parathyroid hormone (hyperplasia). The disease is detected by a raised level of calcium in the blood and urine. The bones appear osteoporotic with loss of bone mineral. Bone resorption may then be noted on radiographs, particularly in the terminal phalanges of the hands and medial aspects of proximal phalanges. This may be shown by using macroradiography. Vascular calcification is also seen and in advanced stages the matrix is replaced by cysts and fibrous tissue. This condition is called osteitis fibrosa cystica or Von Reckinghausen's disease of bone.

The bones also become soft, deformed and prone to damage and bleeding. These cystic, haemorrhagic areas are known as 'brown tumours' and are common in the mandible and pelvis.

Secondary

This form of hyperparathyroidism is caused by chronic renal failure. Chronic renal failure produces a decrease in the blood calcium level that stimulates the parathyroid gland to over-secrete in an attempt to mobilize the calcium present in the bone tissue. This gives rise to demineralization, rickets and osteomalacia. Rarefaction of the vertebral bodies may take place producing the 'rugger jersey' spine.

Brown tumours are rarer, and cyst formation is uncommon in secondary hyperparathyroidism.

Generalized increase in bone density (osteosclerosis)

Causes

Osteopetrosis (marble bone disease, Albers Schönberg's disease)

This is an inherited disease in which the cancellous bone and bone marrow spaces fail to form. This makes the bones very dense because they are composed of a high proportion of compact bone. The bones are hard and brittle and therefore liable to fracture. On the radiograph the bones are seen as dense and structureless because there is little, if any, differentiation between the cortex and medulla of the bone. Anaemia is also found in osteopetrosis. The medulla is underdeveloped and lacking in haemopoietic tissue. This causes the appearance of immature white and red blood cells in the bloodstream together with anaemia (leuco-erythroblastic anaemia).

Myelosclerosis (myelofibrosis)

This involves a replacement of the bone marrow by cancellous bone or fibrous tissue. This results in leuco-erythroblastic anaemia. As the bone becomes increasingly sclerotic the spleen and liver usually take over the sole production of blood cells. This produces splenomegaly which can be seen on radiographs and ultrasound together with generalized patchy sclerotic bones that become denser as the disease progresses. The disease is treated by blood transfusion and has a poor prognosis.

Paget's disease (osteitis deformans)

Paget's disease is an idiopathic osteosclerosis, and is thought to be of viral origin. It occurs in both sexes and is common in the elderly. It is often an incidental finding as a solitary lesion on routine radiographic examination. As a clinical disease produced by multiple lesions it is uncommon. Some patients may complain of localized pain.

The bones appear unevenly dense on the radiograph. The trabeculae become more pronounced and thickened and the bones always expand in width. These changes are due to the increased osteoclast and osteoblast activity. The osteoclast activity is outweighed by the increased osteoblast activity. This produces a bizzare bone structure with islands of new bone isolated by areas of fibrous tissue. These fibrous areas are extremely vascular, which in severe cases may lead to cardiac enlargement as the heart tries to compensate for the increase in size of the body's circulation. Blood tests taken from patients with Paget's disease show normal levels of calcium in the blood and urine although increased blood calcium (hypercalcaemia) may be found in patients who are immobilized following fracture injuries. These fractures are usually incomplete and are called infractions.

Paget's disease is seen throughout the skeleton but most commonly in the skull, vertebral bodies and pelvis. In the skull the disease may be seen as a diffuse patchiness in its early stages, called osteoporosis circumscripta. This will later lead to the bone expansion and an irregular increased trabecular pattern. The outline of the vault is much denser and thickening of the skull base may produce nerve compression and basilar invagination at the foramen magnum.

Replacement by fibrous tissue causes the bones to become very soft. If Paget's disease develops in the vertebrae this may lead to shortening of the spine, kyphosis and a subsequent loss of height. Paget's disease is also common in the pelvis and may often affect only one-half of the pelvic ring. In approximately 1 per cent of cases malignant degeneration of the bone occurs resulting in osteosarcoma.

Paget's disease produces appearances very similar to those found with bony metastatic deposits. However, the two are generally differentiated by the bone expansion found in Paget's disease but absent in secondary deposits.

Treatment of Paget's disease is with injections of thyrocalcitonin or oral disphosphonates which relieve any pain that is present. Treatment is continued for long intervals and may arrest the disease.

Other causes

Other diseases producing localized increase in bone density include:

(1) Sarcoidosis. This is seen in the hands and feet as a mixture of sclerotic and cystic areas.
(2) Bone infarction. Areas of dead bone tissue produce dense sclerotic areas.
(3) Blood disorders. Many blood diseases, e.g. sickle cell anaemia, produce sclerotic areas of bone.
(4) Bone metastases.

Infections

Acute Osteomyelitis

This most commonly affects children. It is caused by *Staphylococcus aureus* or *pyogenes,* although any pyogenic organism can cause osteomyelitis. The organism is usually blood-borne from an area of infection, such as a wound or compound fracture of the bone. Acute osteomyelitis in children occurs most commonly at the metaphysis of the long bones of the lower limbs which is a region that is readily traumatized.

At first the bacteria produce a very localized inflammation. The early stages of the disease are not visible on radiographs. Changes are not usually seen until the infection has been established for approximately ten days.

The infection usually spreads outwards from the medullary cavity, spreading up the medulla or passing outwards through the cortical bone. This causes inflammation of the periosteum (which is seen as characteristic raised area on the radiograph). Bone necrosis and pus formation occur, which accelerates the disease process causing widespread necrosis. A fragment of the bone dies, or, in extreme cases, the whole shaft. This fragment appears very dense and is called a sequestrum. It prevents the drainage of pus away from the site of the disease and thus furthers more chronic disease. This stage is usually classified as the end of the acute phase, but one further stage is often included which involves the formation of a thick bony casing around the sequestrum. This is an attempt at reconstruction of the bone shaft by the periosteum. The result is an imperfect structure that simply retains the pus around the shaft which then leaks through the wall of the involcrum via small sinuses. These will also track up through the muscles and skin surface to form external sinuses.

The disease presents with raised temperature and localized inflammation that is extremely painful. Blood tests reveal the presence of micro-organisms and a rise in the white cell count. Early stages of the disease are well treated by antibiotics. The affected limb is often immobilized in a splint. If the disease is not contained it becomes complicated by pathological fractures, suppurative arthritis and, in extremely virulent infections, death.

Chronic osteomyelitis

This is common in adults, but may be found in children following acute episodes of the disease. The disease develops at a much slower pace than the acute type of the disease. It tends to remain localized to areas of bone rather than spreading throughout the bone shaft. The disease results from localized trauma, i.e. at a fracture site, or may result from surgery to the bone. The infection is caused by *Staphylococcus pyogenes* although other organisms also cause the disease.

Sequestra may be seen in the infected areas of bone or regions of bone destruction. Brodie's abscess may also be seen as a lucent area surrounded by sclerotic bone. Chronic sinus formation is also common.

The condition presents with bouts of fever intermingled with quiescent periods. This may continue for many years.

Chronic osteomyelitis is also treated by antibiotics although the disease is often difficult to cure completely. Surgical drainage may also be carried out, or opening of the medullary cavity to take out the heavily infected bone. In some cases, amputation may be the only course of action to control the infection.

Bone tuberculosis

The bone may become infected from a tuberculous lesion elsewhere in the body, most commonly the lungs. The disease is carried in the bloodstream and most commonly affects the young. The lesion is most often seen in the spine or long bones as destruction and rarefaction of the bone tissue. The bones become softened and liable to pathological fractures.

Congenital diseases

This section is concerned with the changes in bone shape and size that are associated with some congenital abnormalities. Other congenital bone disorders include osteopetrosis and osteogenesis imperfecta.

Achondroplasia

This is a congenital disease of dominant inheritance. It produces shortening of the long bones and therefore dwarfism. The spine and the skull are also affected. The vertebrae become wedge-shaped and narrower than normal when viewed in the antero-posterior projection leading to spinal stenosis. Growth of the base of the skull is arrested prematurely which causes the head to appear disproportionately large. The pelvis is reduced in size and the acetabula are broad and flattened. Overall the bones appear shortened and dense. The disease is caused by an abnormality of the epiphyseal plate. Maturation of the bone takes place very slowly which causes lack of bone growth.

Dyschondroplasia

This type of congenital abnormality is again caused by a defect at the epiphyseal line which results in persistence of cartilage. The cartilage appears as islands of unossified bone among the growing bone. The areas of cartilage (enchondromas) grow and cause expansion of the bone. The condition is commonly found in the hands (Ollier's disease). This may result in loss of function in some cases and may need to be treated by extensive surgery to regain some use of the fingers. In some cases of dyschondroplasia cancellous spurs topped with cartilage may grow away from the affected epiphyseal line. These ecchondromas or exostoses are most common at the knee joint and may be palpable through the skin. This condition is called diaphyseal aclasia or multiple exostoses, which occasionally form chondrosarcoma.

Gigantism and acromegaly

Both conditions are produced by over-secretion of growth hormone by the anterior pituitary gland. This is most commonly due to the presence of an adenoma in the anterior pituitary. Adenomas are simple endocrine glands formed from regular symmetrical cells.

If increased secretion of growth hormone takes place before fusion of the epiphysis then there is a uniform increase in bone growth producing a well-proportioned giant (gigantism).

Following epiphyseal union increased excretion of growth hormone results in acromegaly. This is characterized by increased growth of the hands and feet, and overgrowth of the jaw. The skull vault also thickens and the pituitary fossa is generally enlarged and eroded by the presence of the adenoma.

Skin thickness also increases in acromegaly and may be used to detect and follow the course of the disease. Measuring the thickness of tissues around the calcaneum was once taken as an indication of the disease. This 'heel pad thickness' is measured from true lateral soft tissue projections of the heel. This system is now not commonly used and levels of growth hormone are now more reliably assessed from radio-immuno-assay of blood samples.

Tumours of bone

Radiographically it is often very difficult to identify a bone tumour, and it is often the underlying medical history that identifies the lesion. For example, it is sometimes difficult to differentiate osteomyelitis from bone tumour. The two are separated by the presence of a sinus, generally only found in osteomyelitis, or by previous radiographs that may confirm the presence of a small bone tumour. Generally, acute osteomyelitis is quick to develop as opposed to most bone tumours. Primary bone tumours are comparatively uncommon. Secondary bone tumours are much more common.

Bone, and other related tumours are classified by their tissue of origin. Thus a chondroma arises from cartilage. As with other connective tissue tumours the suffix *-oma* implies benign and *-sarcoma* malignant. All bone tumours arise from osteoblasts (Figure 11.3).

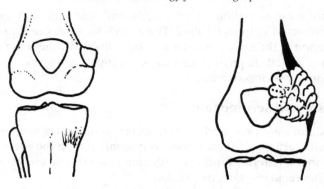

Figure 11.3 Types of bone tumour: osteoma (left) and osteosarcoma (right)

Osteoma

This is a benign tumour of bone. Osteoma may be seen as bony outgrowths near to joints and particularly the knee joint. In some cases the osteoma may become malignant and form an osteosarcoma (below). If the outgrowth becomes painful then it may be excised.

Osteosarcoma (osteogenic sarcoma)

This is a primary malignant tumour of bone tissue. It commonly occurs in patients between the ages of ten and twenty-five years and is more common in males. When found in older patients it is usually associated with Paget's disease. The tumour usually occurs at the ends of long bones and is commonest in the femur, particularly around the knee joint. The lesion is also found in the tibia and proximal humerus. The underlying cause of the disease is not understood.

The tumour is very aggressive and usually grows from the metaphysis, destroying both the medulla and cortex. The tumour is very vascular and composed of deformed osteoblasts that give rise to a mixture of tissue types. New bone formation may take place and flecks of new bone may be seen within the tumour. The tumour generally breaks through to the periosteum causing a severe periosteal reaction. The periosteum becomes raised and produces a triangular outgrowth of periosteal tissue called 'Codman's triangle'. This sign is not specific to osteosarcoma and may be seen in many other lesions.

The tumour is found on radiographs taken following pain in a limb not obviously associated with trauma. On discovery the lesion is quickly biopsied and confirmation of the disease usually results in amputation of the limb and treatment with cytotoxic drugs. Bone scans will be taken in a search for secondary spread. Spread of the tumour is usually by a vascular route to the lungs, or in fewer cases by the lymphatic system.

Osteoblastoma

This is a rare benign tumour of the young. The lesion is generally found in the neural arch and is characterized by expansion of the bone. In the spinal column this results in spinal cord compression and is therefore dangerous in this respect rather than for its secondary effects.

Tumours of cartilage

Chondroma

This is a benign tumour of cartilage. It is subdivided into two types:

(1) Ecchondroma which forms cartilagenous outgrowths in diaphyseal aclasia.
(2) Enchondroma found as persistent areas of cartilage that cause bony expansion in the condition of dyschondroplasia.

Chondrosarcoma

This is a primary malignant tumour of cartilage cells (chondroblasts). The tumour occurs in the young, i.e. under the age of twenty-five and is commoner in men. It is found in the long bones, the pelvis and scapulae. The tumour is very slow-growing and may not cause any detectable symptoms. The tumour may arise from an underlying ecchondroma and is seen as an expanded area of cystic-like bone on radiographs.

The lesion will eventually metastasise via the blood and lymphatic system. Treatment is as radical as with osteosarcoma, requiring amputation and treatment with cytotoxic drugs. There is a 50 per cent five-year survival rate. Disruption of the tumour on removal lowers the survival rate due to the formation of secondaries.

Chondroblastoma (Codman's tumour)

This is a rare benign tumour of the chondroblasts. It occurs in adolescents and grows out from the epiphyseal region of the bone, and is commonly found in the proximal humerus. It is usually treated by excision to prevent possible malignancy.

Fibrous tumours of bone

Fibroma of bone

This is a rare, benign tumour of bone. The lesion presents as a well-defined lucent area and may be found by chance while radiographing other regions. It may be resected if it causes problems, but often recurs.

Fibrosarcoma of bone

This malignant primary fibrous tumour occurs in young adults. The tumour metastasises via the blood and lymphatic system. It grows quickly and requires surgical removal. Fibrosarcomas of periosteal origin, if removed, have a 25 per cent, five-year survival rate.

Osteoclastoma (giant-cell tumour)

This is a primary bone tumour of the osteoclasts. Osteoclastomas occur as eccentric expanding tumours at the end of long bones. The knee and wrist are the most common sites. It expands slowly and a tumour with well-defined margins forms. The tumour gains its name from the large osteoclast-like cells it contains. Giant cell tumours are locally invasive but may metastasise via the bloodstream usually to the lungs. The tumour is treated by complete surgical removal or amputation of the affected area of bone.

Tumours of bone marrow

Ewing's tumour

This is a highly malignant primary tumour that occurs in red bone marrow and is therefore most common in children and teenagers. However it may be found in the bones of adults containing red marrow, e.g. pelvis and scapulae. The tumour produces widespread bone destruction and formation of new bone in the periosteum. This new bone may form multiple layers giving a characteristic onion skin appearance. Codman's triangle may also be seen.

The tumour is very malignant and metastasises quickly via the bloodstream. Pulmonary secondaries are common and the disease is nearly always fatal. Fever and pain are associated with the tumour and treatment is by radical radiotherapy.

Myeloma

This is a relatively common malignant disease of the bone marrow. More specifically it is a tumour affecting the plasma cells that produce the immunoglobulins (antibodies). Myeloma is described as a proliferative disease, and thus there is an over-production of immunoglobulin. Antibodies are large protein-based molecules and therefore a patient with myeloma will show an increase of blood proteins. The disease may be confirmed by electropheresis of the blood serum which will show raised levels of immunoglobulin particularly IgG. Other abnormal proteins may also be produced, e.g. Bence Jones protein which occurs in approximately 65 per cent of cases. This is detected in the urine of affected patients.

Myeloma is a disease found mainly in the elderly. When detected it is usually found as multiple lytic areas (myelomatosis) in bones with active haemopoiesis, e.g. ribs, pelvis, humerus. The disease presents on radiographs as lytic lesions spread throughout the skeleton. The appearance may mimic secondary deposits (see below). Therefore the disease is confirmed by the presence of unusual proteins in the blood and urine and excessive plasma cells in the bone marrow. Bone marrow samples and bone scans show the extent of the disease. Single isolated lesions are rare. The disease is associated with anaemia and pathological fractures and is treated primarily by chemotherapy using cyclophosphamide. Back-up therapy such as renal dialysis may also be given.

Leukaemia

See pp. 83–87.

Other tumours associated with bone

(1) Lipoma. Benign soft tissue tumour.
(2) Liposarcoma. Rare, very malignant, tumour requiring excision of affected tissue.
(3) Haemangiomas. Vascular malformations.
(4) Neurofibroma. This tumour of nerve tissue is rare in bone.

Secondary bone tumours

These are by far the most common bone tumours. Bones with active haemopoiesis are more liable to secondary deposits. Tumours that most frequently metastasise to bone are carcinomas of the breast, bronchus, kidney, prostate, stomach and thyroid. Leukaemias and lymphomas also give rise to secondaries. The size and extent of the bone lesions varies enormously, most producing localized bone destruction. A periosteal reaction may also be seen.

Sclerotic secondaries are seen with prostatic and breast carcinomas. Secondary deposits are the most frequent cause of pathological fractures. Pathological fractures are actively treated by orthopaedic surgery.

Bone cysts

These are benign lesions and when large cause bone expansion and bone weakness. This results in pathological fractures in some cases. These lesions are common in children. On radiographs the cyst presents as a lucent cavity surrounded by a thin complete shell. The cavity is fluid filled. A variant is the aneurysmal bone cyst in which the cavity fills with blood due to arteriovenous malformation within the bone cavity. The lesion is treated by excision or by radiotherapy.

THE JOINTS

Normal anatomy of the synovial joint can be seen in Figure 11.4.

(1) The articular surfaces of the bones forming the joint are covered in hyaline cartilage. Hyaline cartilage is avascular and receives nutrients from the synovial fluid. The joint surfaces may be separated by pads of fibrocartilage, e.g. the knee joint where the pads are called menisci.

(2) There is a joint cavity between the articular surfaces that contains the synovial fluid.

(3) The joint is surrounded by a fibrous capsule called the articular capsule.

(4) Synovial membrane covers the surface of the joint except the articular cartilage and secretes the synovial fluid. The synovial membrane may give rise to bursae lying outside the joint.

(5) The joint capsule is strengthened by ligaments.

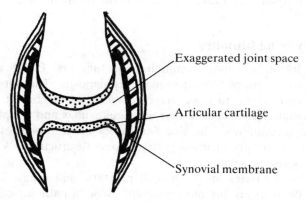

Exaggerated joint space

Articular cartilage

Synovial membrane

Figure 11.4   Synovial joint

(6) A wide range of movement occurs at synovial joints.
(7) The joint receives nerve and blood supply.

Most of the joint disease described below involves synovial joints.

Diseases affecting children
Congenital dislocation of the hip (CDH)

Screening for CDH at birth is common practice. The baby is placed supine and both legs are abducted as far as possible in an attempt to dislocate the hip. If the hip appears stiff and dislocates then the child has a CDH. In this manoeuvre the hips may be heard to click when the hip is reduced. This is a characteristic of children with CDH.

The child is not usually radiographed until three months old. It is very difficult to interpret the radiographs before this age as the bone is still immature. If the child is radiographed then this is carried out with the child's legs in the true AP position. It is essential that the pelvis is perfectly symmetrical when viewed on the finished radiograph.

The radiograph appearances in the neonate may appear normal. In older children, and especially those who have began to bear weight, the acetabulum will appear flattened when compared to the normal pelvis of a similarly aged child.

If the CDH is not detected at birth then the child will begin to walk with a waddle. A radiograph of children at this stage will show deformities of the joint capsule. Arthrography of the hip is often carried out under general anaesthetic to show the extent and site of the deformity.

The cause of CDH is not understood although the condition is due to a lax hip joint. A variety of factors are associated with the disease. For instance, CDH is more common with breech births and an increased incidence of CDH is noted if another member of the family was born with the condition.

If the CDH is detected at birth then the condition is treated by putting the babies into double nappies to hold the femoral head in correct relation to the acetabulum, but if the CDH is not detected at birth, and is detected before the child walks, then the dislocation is reduced by placing the child in bed traction. This is followed up by keeping the legs in a plaster cast. The plaster and associated splinting will usually hold the legs abducted and in external rotation.

Should arthrography of the hip reveal deformities of the acetabulum or joint capsule, then surgical intervention may be necessary. This ranges from removal of a trapped portion of the joint capsule to rebuilding the acetabulum with a bone graft (pelvic osteotomy).

Children with undetected or late treated CDH show a greater incidence of arthritic changes on adulthood.

Osteochondritis

Osteochondritis is a disease of epiphyseal bone prior to fusion. The term refers to a number of diseases each with the same underlying pathological features. The disease is associated with repeated trauma to the affected bone and associated joint. The trauma results in an interrupted blood supply and death of the bone tissue (avascular necrosis). Radiographs of the affected bones show areas of sclerosis, deformity of the bone and attempts at remodelling through callus formation. The lesion occurs in many sites but is commonest in the hip.

Perthes' disease

This is osteochondritis of the upper femoral epiphysis (Figure 11.5). The condition is more common in boys. In some cases it is bilateral. The cause is thought to be related to injury and presents as a pain in the hip with pain on weight-bearing. The pain develops over some time and may be detected on radiograph following a sporting injury.

On radiography of the hip epiphysis may appear as though it were in small fragments. Cysts may develop in the femoral neck and the metaphysis may appear widened. As the disease progresses, the bone will form callus and remodel. This frequently leaves the head flattened and distorted when seen on follow-up radiographs. Frequently lateral projections are taken to show the extent of the damage of the femoral head. It is essential that good early projections of both hips are taken because early detection of the disease gives a much better chance of recovery.

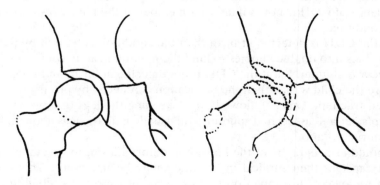

Figure 11.5   Perthes' disease: unaffected hip joint (left) and affected hip (right)

Treatment of the condition is frequently conservative. This may involve putting the child on traction with the hip in internal rotation and abduction. This will hold the hip in the acetabulum and mould it to its normal shape. However, if the epiphysis becomes prone to subluxation (partial dislocation), then surgical intervention may be required. This may involve an osteotomy to the acetabulum. A portion of bone is added to the acetabulum to prevent the hip subluxing.

Other forms of osteochondritis

Osgood-Schlatter's disease

This is osteochondritis of the tibial tubercle. It is commonest in boys and frequently bilateral. The tubercle becomes fragmented with inflammation of the surrounding tissue. The patient presents with localized pain at the tibial tubercle. Lateral radiographs of both knees must be taken. The disease rarely needs treatment.

Kohler's disease

Osteochondritis of the navicular bone.

Kienböck's disease

Osteochondritis of the lunate bone.

Sever's disease

Osteochondritis of the calcaneum.

Frieberg's disease

Osteochondritis of the heads of the metatarsals.

Osteochondritis dissecan

This is a very localized form of osteochondritis, affecting very small areas of bone. It is most common in the knee joint. The area of affected bone detaches from the underlying healthy bone and floats loose within the joint cavity. The patient presents with pain and tenderness in the joint. The knee may also lock or click. Intercondylar views of the knee will confirm the presence of a loose body. The knee may be strapped and immobilized until the pain subsides. In some cases the fragment may be removed to prevent infection of the joint.

Slipped femoral epiphysis

This is a condition that occurs following trauma. However the condition may occur spontaneously particularly in overweight children. The condition has been associated with a hormonal imbalance. It is commoner in boys and it is bilateral in approximately 25 per cent of all patients.

The child presents with pain in the hip and on the radiograph the femoral epiphysis is seen to have slipped posteriorly. Thus a true lateral projection of the hip will best demonstrate the lesion. The limb will appear difficult to internally rotate.

The condition is managed by placing the child on traction in internal rotation which holds the epiphysis in position. If the slip cannot be stabilized by traction, then the epiphysis will be pinned in position by passing three pins through the neck of the femur into the femoral head. Following pinning the patient will be kept on traction and the pins will be removed when the femoral head has stabilized and the epiphysis has fused.

Adult and generalized diseases

Avascular necrosis

As we have seen (p. 258), osteochondritis manifests itself in many different sites of the body with very little explanation of the cause. However, there are many other conditions that also cause avascular necrosis. These include:

(1) Fractures. Avascular necrosis of the scaphoid may occur following fracture of the body of the bone (see p. 286).
(2) Caisson's disease (decompression sickness). This occurs in people who have work in increased atmospheric pressures, e.g. deep sea divers. If return to the surface pressure is too quick dissolved gases in the bloodstream come out of the blood in the form of bubbles ('the bends'). The oxygen and carbon dioxide formed are quickly resorbed while any nitrogen bubbles formed remain in the bloodstream. Bones and joints are most susceptible to these nitrogen emboli and if untreated cause necrosis of the bone ends and subsequent loss of the articular surfaces. Thus divers often have their knees and shoulders radiographed to detect any early changes in their joints.
(3) Steroids. Long-term use of steroids may also cause bone and joint necrosis.

Inflammatory joint disease

Rheumatoid arthritis

This is a chronic inflammatory disease of connective tissue which usually affects the joints. The disease is more common in women. Its cause is unknown, but there are a number of suspected causes. These include viruses and bacteria, genetic factors and endocrine problems. The patient presents with pain in one or more joints associated with swelling and joint stiffness. As the disease enters its chronic stage the joints become very swollen, inflamed and fluid-filled.

Radiographs of early rheumatoid arthritis show soft tissue swelling and osteoporosis around the joints. These changes may be quite subtle and thus macroradiographs of the hands and wrists may be taken to show early disease. In later stages of the disease the changes are marked by widespread destruction of the bone ends around the joints, and gross deformities.

The disease may also be detected by blood tests. RA or rheumatoid arthritis factor is found in 90 per cent of cases with rheumatoid arthritis. RA factor is an antibody (IgM) that attacks and attaches to non-active or foreign IgG, and so is used as the basis for the latex test. Latex particles are coated with human or rabbit IgG and the effect of the rheumatoid blood on the IgG is noted. RA factor will bind with the IgG. Other similar methods are also used.

Connective tissue is widespread in the body. Thus rheumatoid arthritis is found in many different systems. The spine may become deformed or fused and subluxation of the atlanto-axial joint may take place as the odontoid peg moves forward. This is demonstrated on flexion and extension views. The skin and muscle are also affected. The skin appears papery and there is inflammation of the muscles including the heart. Lung tissue may also be affected together with the blood vessels. The rheumatoid patient often presents as a frail old lady with weight loss and difficulty in walking.

The disease is treated with salicylates, e.g. aspirin, which both relieve pain and reduce inflammation. Steroids may be used in some cases, but these are known to cause osteoporosis if used over long periods. Surgery may also be used, ranging from joint fusion to removal of affected tendons and the use of joint prostheses.

Rheumatoid arthritis is a crippling disease and patients often need a lot of support from family and friends to help them cope with the deformities of hands and feet that the disease can bring. Home visits are often carried out by occupational therapists to assess the patients in the home environment. Physiotherapy may also be used to help free the stiffness that develops in the diseased joints.

Remission from the disease does take place, but is usually only temporary. The deformities always remain unless surgically corrected. The disease is often complicated by osteoarthritis and polyarteritis nodosa which causes diffuse inflammation and destruction of the walls of arteries throughout the vascular system.

Still's disease (juvenile rheumatoid arthritis)

This is much less common than the adult form of the disease. The disease may be of slow onset or associated with episodes of fever. The main joints affected are the knee, ankle and wrist. Radiographs of the joints may show no change in the early stages as with the adult form of the disease. Osteoporosis occurs in later stages and premature fusion of the epiphysis may take place. The child is generally treated the same as the adult. Still's disease shows a much higher recovery rate than adult rheumatoid arthritis.

Reiter's disease

This uncommon disease is thought to be of bacterial origin. The disease causes urethritis and conjunctivitis and is a type of atypical rheumatoid arthritis of the joints. The disease is not as widespread as classical rheumatoid arthritis.

Ankylosing spondylitis

This is a rare condition and is found predominantly in young males between the ages of fifteen and thirty-five. The disease is usually restricted to the lumbar spine and starts with inflammation of the ligaments of the spine. This leads to fibrous replacement and calcification of the ligaments and the intervertebral discs. The spine becomes rigid and has the characteristic 'bamboo spine' appearance when viewed on radiographs. The disease, by this point, has invariably spread to include the sacroiliac joints and upwards to the neck.

The patient presents with back pain and stiffness that may have been of long standing.

Treatment is usually conservative. Physiotherapy may be given to patients with difficulty in bending and movement to prevent fixed flexion and other spinal deformities. Analgesia is given if the patient has pain.

Gout

This is another form of arthritis but is not related to rheumatoid disease. Gout is a metabolic disease that results from poor purine metabolism. The caffeine found in tea and coffee is a purine derivative that, at its final stage of breakdown, forms uric acid (2,6,8 trihydoxy-purine). In gout uric acid is retained in the bloodstream which causes deposition of uric acid as sodium mono-urate crystals in the joints. This causes severe joint pain and swelling. The joint becomes red and painful on movement and the disease is usually restricted to one joint. The attack will stop after a few days but will probably recur if the disease is not controlled. Repeated attacks will cause extensive bone damage due to the deposition of the urate crystals. In more advanced cases urates are deposited in the skin to form small swollen areas around the joints called tophi. These areas may calcify.

The urate crystals in the joint and adjacent bones gives rise to osteoarthritis. This is most commonly seen in men and is generally seen around the metatarsophalangeal joint of the big toe. Radiographs may show soft tissue swelling and erosion of the joint together with osteophyte production. The bony erosions may be at some distance from the site of the joint, which distinguishes gout from other forms of arthritis. Tophi may also be seen as calcified lesions.

The disease is triggered by alcohol and rich foods and is detected and monitored by measuring the levels of uric acid in the blood and urine. Treatment is by drugs that lower the uric acid level of the blood, e.g. indomethacin. If poorly managed, or if the patient is in poor health, gout can lead to renal failure and other complications. As the disease progresses many joints become infected.

Calcification of the articular cartilage with crystals of calcium pyrophosphate is called pseudogout or crystal synovitis.

Suppurative arthritis

This type of arthritis is caused by blood-borne infection, e.g. *Staphylococcus aureus*. This may be as a result of osteomyelitis (pyogenic arthritis). Suppurative arthritis associated with osteomyelitis is more common in children. The child experiences acute pain as the joint becomes pus-filled. Erosion of the joint follows with destruction of the articular cartilage. If the disease continues granular tissue replaces the cartilage. This tissue organizes itself to produce fibrous tissue that results in joint fusion (ankylosis). Fibrous ankylosis will be replaced by complete bone fusion of the joint.

On radiography early changes will not be seen, but as the disease progresses bony changes and soft tissue swelling will be seen. The disease is diagnosed by aspirating the affected joint and analysing the pus for evidence of bacteria. The condition is treated by antibiotics and, in some cases, surgical drainage of the joint.

Tuberculosis is caused by the bacteria *Mycobacterium tuberculosis*. Tubercule infection of joints causes changes similar to rheumatoid arthritis. The two are differentiated by the widespread osteoporosis shown by joints that are infected by tuberculosis. Spread is usually from a pulmonary lesion or other isolated lesions. Infection of joints and vertebrae of the spine is called Pott's disease.

Osteoarthritis

This is the most common form of arthritis. It is extremely common amongst the elderly but may occur in younger patients following trauma to the limbs.

If the disease is related to a previous injury or trauma then it is termed secondary. Primary osteoarthritis has no obvious cause. The disease is thought to be a result of wear and tear on the joints and bones although disruption of collagen metabolism is also suspected, i.e. breakdown of connective tissue. Osteoarthritis most commonly occurs in the weight-bearing joints, e.g. the knees and hips.

The covering of articular cartilage erodes away and the underlying bone takes the weight of the limb. This causes extra bone to grow. The extra bone is seen as outgrowths (osteophytes) on the side of the bone. This also results in narrowing of the joint space and formation of cysts under the bone surface. Sclerosis at the bone ends is also common due to the increased weight-bearing taken up by the limb. On radiographs this will be seen as a dense white line on either side of the joint. Occasionally loose bodies will be seen within the joint space. Weight-bearing radiographs are usually taken to show the extent of the joint narrowing and the extent of the limb deformity that takes place in advanced cases.

The disease is treated with analgesics to relieve joint pain and physiotherapy to relieve joint stiffness. The disease is not as acute as rheumatoid arthritis.

Artificial joint replacement (arthroplasty) may be carried out. Hip and knee replacements are quite common and with follow-up physiotherapy produce excellent results.

Osteo- and rheumatoid arthritis can be distinguished from each other as follows:

Osteo	Rheumatoid
No osteoporosis	Osteoporosis
Cyst formation	No cysts
Minor bone erosion	Extensive erosions
Chronic	Tends to fairly acute
Little tissue involvement	Pain, swelling
Osteophytes and widespread sclerosis	Few osteophytes

Neuropathic arthritis (Charcot joints)

This is an extreme form of joint degeneration due to the loss of sensory nerve supply to the joint. The disease is most commonly found in the knee and hip joint due to spinal lesions such as tales dorsalis or syringomyelia.

The affected joint shows large effusions and rapid instability. The joint literally falls apart while the patient is unaware of any pain. Diabetics also suffer from this condition in advanced cases and radiographs of the feet may reveal extensive fractures and widespread calcification.

12
FRACTURES

A fracture is either a complete break in the continuity of a bone or an incomplete break or crack. Fractures can be broadly divided into three groups:

(1) Fractures caused by sudden, abrupt injury. These fractures form the largest group and can occur in bones that are free from disease. Fractures of this type may be caused by direct violence, e.g. road traffic accident (RTA), or indirect violence.
(2) Stress or fatigue fractures. These occur in bones under often repeated stress and not from a direct blow. Their aetiology is often unknown and they have been likened to the structural fatigue found in various metals after long usage. The majority of stress fractures are confined to the lower limb. Most occur in the metatarsals but others can be seen in the shaft of the fibula and tibia and neck of the femur.
(3) Pathological fractures. A fracture is classed as pathological when the bone has already been weakened by disease. The fracture may occur spontaneously or from minimal trauma.

CATEGORIES

Fractures (Figure 12.1) are described either by the way the fracture took place (see Pott's fracture, p. 291) or by the shape or pattern of the fracture surface (e.g. the oblique fracture). The pattern and description of the fracture are useful to the clinician when reducing or re-aligning the fracture. It may also indicate the stability of the fragments.

The following terms are in general use when describing categories of fracture:

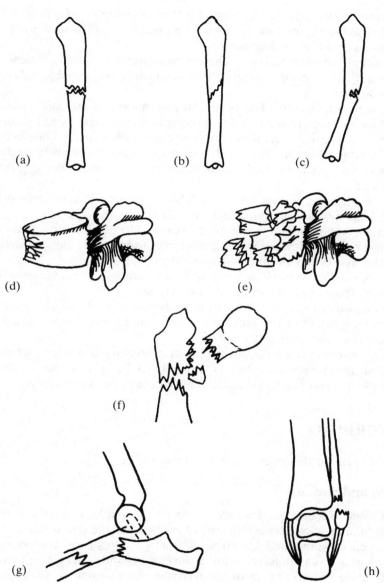

Figure 12.1   Types of fracture: (a) transverse; (b) oblique or spiral; (c) greenstick;
(d) compression; (e) burst; (f) comminuted; (g) fracture dislocation
and (h) avulsion fracture

(1) Transverse fracture. This type of fracture is caused by direct violence. A transverse fracture is unlikely to become redisplaced following re-alignment of the fragments.

(2) Oblique or spiral fracture. This is often caused by twisting strains and is a typical sporting injury. This is much more unstable following reduction.

(3) Greenstick fracture. This occurs only in children. The bone bends and does not fracture completely, the cortex on the concave side remaining intact. Alternatively, if longitudinal compression of the bone occurs, the bone takes on a crumpled, folded appearance. Complete fractures may also occur in children, although they are rarer than greenstick fractures.

(4) Compression or crush fractures. This is common in cancellous bone, e.g. spongy bone as found in the vertebral column.

(5) Burst fracture. This is the most extreme form of fracture. It usually occurs in short bones causing extensive disruption to bone structure. This may be as a result of a road accident.

(6) Avulsion fracture. Usually caused by a tendon or ligament tearing off a bony fragment and may be difficult to reduce.

(7) Fracture dislocation is a fracture involving a joint. It usually results in mal-alignment of the joint space, and may require surgical intervention, i.e. and 'open reduction'.

(8) Comminuted fractures. A comminuted fracture is made up of more than two fragments. This, as with a burst fracture, is due to severe violence, and union of the fragments is both difficult and delayed.

DESCRIPTION

Fractures can be described by the following terms:

Open and closed

(1) Closed fracture. A fracture is closed or simple when there is no communication between the site of fracture and the skin surface.

(2) Open or compound fractures. A fracture is open or 'compounded' when it communicates with a surface wound. Thus a transverse fracture of the tibia with an overlying open wound is a compound fracture.

Complicated

If, as a result of a fracture, nerve damage or damage to other vessels occurs then the fracture is called complicated. One example is the supracondylar fracture of the humerus. Both the median and ulnar nerves and blood supply to the hand may be severed by the forward movement of the fracture fragments.

Impacted

When all the fracture fragments are driven into each other, the fracture is said to be impacted. This type is usually stable as opposed to a comminuted fracture which is classified as unstable.

FRACTURES IN CHILDREN

In addition to greenstick fractures, children may also sustain epiphyseal injuries (Figure 12.2). Epiphyseal fractures may be classified into five categories (Salter and Harrison):

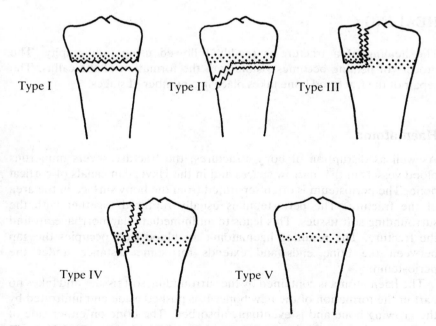

Figure 12.2 Fractures in children (Salter and Harris classification)

Type I. The fracture line passes clearly through the epiphyseal line but produces no metaphyseal fragments. This type occurs in young children or neonates and may be associated with pathological conditions such as vitamin C deficiency or spina bifida.

Type II. The fracture line runs, at first, across the epiphyseal line and then obliquely shears off small triangular fragments of metaphysis. This is the most common type.

Type III. The fracture line passes vertically through the epiphysis and a fragment displaces along the line of the epiphysis.

Type IV. The fracture line extends through the epiphyseal line into the metaphysis. This type may interfere with growth because union may take place across the displaced growth plate also causing mal-alignment of the bone. Premature fusion of the epiphysis may be avoided by open reduction and internal fixation.

Type V. Compression fracture of the epiphysis. This type results in arrest of growth and deformity of the bone. Type V has a poor prognosis because it is often missed on initial examination.

HEALING

The healing of a fracture is readily followed using radiography. The process of healing becomes visible with the formation of the callus. The repair of the fractured bone takes place in a number of stages.

Haematoma

As well as disruption of bony structures, the fracture severs numerous blood vessels in the marrow spaces and in the Haversian canals of cortical bone. The periosteum is often separated from the bony surface in the area of the fracture. The periosteum is usually ruptured together with the surrounding soft tissues. This leads to an immediate haemorrhage around the fracture. The resulting haematoma, or blood clot, occupies the gap between the bone ends and extends for some distance under the periosteum.

The haematoma is contained by the surrounding soft tissues and takes no part in the formation of the new bone. It is pushed aside and infiltrated by the growing bone and is eventually absorbed. The bone on either side of the fracture becomes ischaemic over a varying length.

Subperiosteal and endosteal proliferation

The tissue damage resulting from the fracture acts as a stimulus to osteoblast activity and there is a proliferation in the number of osteoblasts at the fracture site. The growth of the rapidly forming osteoblasts takes place between the ends of the fracture, their growth being sustained by the network of blood vessels that grows throughout the haematoma. Islands of cartilage or chondroblasts may also be seen at this stage growing between the bone tissues, forming a bridge between the bone ends.

Callus formation

The tissue lying between the bones now begins to mature. This stage begins at approximately six to ten weeks. Osteoblasts continue to form at the fracture site. The osteoblasts lay down a matrix of collagen and polysaccharides that, together with calcium, form an immature woven bone called osteoid tissue or callus. Any cartilage present also matures. Cartilage forms where development of the callus is most rapid, particularly at the surface of the fracture. It is the callus that ultimately establishes bony continuity between the fractured bones. The amount of callus varies, but is present in greater amounts when the fracture is allowed to move slightly. When no movement occurs at the fracture site, little or no callus forms.

Rigid internal fixation, as in the use of a prosthesis or plating to immobilize a fracture, may suppress the formation of callus. Fracture braces and some prostheses allow minimal movement of the fracture site to promote healing.

Consolidation

The woven bone that makes up the primary callus now begins to take on the typical lamellar structure. The fracture becomes less mobile and bone growth continues until ultimately the fracture reaches clinical union. Clinical union of a long bone takes three to four months. Any cartilage present demonstrates the same maturing process as seen in the epiphyseal plate, becoming calcified and converting to endochondral bone. Complete, so-called 'radiological union' may appear much later whereby complete cortex to cortex union can be seen, i.e. a continuation of trabeculae across the site of the fracture.

Fractures in cancellous bone, e.g. the vertebral body, heal more quickly than the average long bone. There is no medullary canal present, therefore union takes place directly between bony surfaces and there is no need for the formation of an intermediate callus. This reduces union time to approximately eight weeks. Union in children's bone occurs more quickly than adult bone, and requires two to three weeks for the average long bone.

Non-union

Sometimes fractures do not heal. Clinically, a fracture is tested to see whether union has taken place by trying to induce movement at the site of the fracture and by noting any signs of pain on manipulation of the affected area. Non-union is a clinical and radiological diagnosis and is infuenced by the appearance of radiographs. The absence of callus is diagnosed as delayed or non-union of the fracture. A number of other factors influence union of fractures:

(1) Age. As indicated above, fracture repair is much faster in children and babies. In old age, other related diseases such as osteoporosis may influence fracture repair and cause fracturing of the femoral neck.

(2) Fracture site. A fracture that involves loss of blood supply to any bone or bony fragment will result in an increase in the time it takes for union to occur.

(3) Infection. Bony infections, e.g. osteomyelitis, delays union of fractures.

(4) Immobilization. Immobilization aids the union of a fracture, adding stability to extensive fractures. However, immobilization will generally prolong the time of healing by precluding the formation of callus.

(5) Extent of fractures. A combination of fractures in a limb, or multiple fractures, will usually increase the length of time of union.

(6) State of health. In vitamin deficiency diseases, e.g. vitamin C deficiency, fracture healing is delayed due to disruption of callus formation. Lack of callus formation is called atrophic non-union.

(7) Hypertrophic non-union. The over-production of callus around the fractured ends of a bone may also preclude satisfactory union.

(8) Excessive movement of the fracture ends delays union.

Treatment of non-union is generally surgical, requiring the application of bone grafts around the site of the fracture. However, electrical stimulation of the fracture site may be used. An alternating or direct current is used that sets up a field within the bone and has been shown to promote callus formation.

Non-union of infected fractures usually requires radical treatment in the form of excision of infected bone, together with bone grafting and antibiotics. This is followed by rigid immobilization of the fracture site. Metal plating is avoided due to the likelihood of reinfection of the fracture site and grafted bone. Thus, interno-external fixation is used, e.g. Steinmann or Fischer-type pins that act as a rigid scaffold around the fracture.

Remodelling

Once union of the fracture is complete and the bone is stable, remodelling of the bone takes place. Remodelling of bone is a continual process that takes place throughout life, being regulated by the stresses and strains exerted on the bone. The changes are minute and mapped out in the trabeculae. Following injury, the process is readily observed.

The amount of bony callus formed, and its distribution, are governed by the way forces act on the fracture site. Bone is deposited where stresses and strains are at their greatest and is removed where it does not have a useful function in providing mechanical strength. The time taken to model the callus such that radiological union is achieved, i.e. a smooth outline to the bone, depends upon the amount of callus present following consolidation. Callus is usually predominant in children's fractures, but remodelling is also very extensive and the point of the fracture is usually difficult to distinguish from native bone following remodelling. The remodelling process is a fine balance between both osteoblasts and osteoclasts re-sculpturing the bone.

Complications

Osteomyelitis

Wound infection usually remains superficial, but may extend down to the bone, giving rise to osteomyelitis. This is an inflammation of areas of bone, i.e. the contents of the medullary cavity and Haversian canals and the periosteum. The calcified portions of the bone take no active part in the disease process but die as a result of loss of blood supply. Prolonged ischaemia may result in death of the bone tissue. An area of dead bone may form a sequestrum that may lie loose within a cavity of the bone unless removed by surgical means. This area of necrotic bone may be accompanied by a discharging sinus.

Skin and soft tissue necrosis

These also accompany osteomyelitis due to lack of blood supply to the superficial tissues due to underlying bone necrosis.

Gangrene

This is an extreme form of cell necrosis. Dry gangrene may appear in a patient who has completely occluded the blood supply to the foot after gross trauma of the tibia. The foot will become pulseless, cold and will have no collateral circulation. Rarely, gangrene and cell death may result from incorrectly applied plaster or tourniquets in the early stages of the treatment of fractures.

Gas gangrene

This is a rare complication of fracture healing and repair that arises as a result of post-operative infection of the wound or through chronically infected wounds. Anaerobic bacteria, e.g. *Clostridium perfringes,* may become lodged in the tissue around the fracture site. The gas is a by-product of bacterial metabolism.

Tetanus

This may appear together with gas gangrene. As with gangrene, tetanus is produced by an anaerobic bacillus, *Clostridium tetani.* Tetanus starts as an infection of a septic wound and produces hypersensitivity of the motor nerve cells. This causes extreme pain and puts the affected area into violent spasm.

Pressure sores

With patients undergoing long periods of traction, pressure sores must be avoided. This is particularly important with the elderly. Attention must be paid to keeping pressure sites clean, especially where turning the patient is prevented by traction.

Deep vein thrombosis and pulmonary embolism

Thrombosis generally occurs in immobilized limbs following long-term traction or use of plaster casts. The thrombus may appear post-operatively but generally develops due to slowing and pooling of the blood and damage to the vessel walls, thus encouraging the formation of clots. Generally the formation of venous clots is associated with other factors such as heart disease.

A pulmonary embolism occurs as a result of thrombus formation in another part of the body. A portion of the thrombus becomes detached (thromboembolism) and is taken into the pulmonary circulation. Should the clot occlude a sizeable branch of the pulmonary artery, death may result. Once again, this generally occurs with patients confined to bed, particularly to people with varicose veins.

Pneumonia

This is an inflammatory consolidation of the lung. It is common in the elderly, where general health tends to be poor.

Fat embolism

This is a little-understood process that may cause severe problems. Fat embolus develops from one to several days following the fracture. It is most common where extensive trauma has taken place. If left untreated, large amounts of fat emboli will become dislodged and pass to the pulmonary circulation and other areas of the body, e.g. kidneys and liver. These fat globules may pass through the pulmonary capillaries and so on to the brain. The patient presents with difficulty in breathing and growing confusion which may result in coma or death.

The origin of the fat is not fully understood. It is thought that following trauma, the normal fat within the bloodstream aggregates together into larger more dangerous amounts.

Fat embolus can be treated by early immobilization of fractures, intensive respiratory care and by giving fluids to the patient, i.e. replacing fluids lost through injury.

'Crush syndrome'

Injury to large areas of tissue following extensive trauma, e.g. RTA, is usually associated with damage and occlusion of major blood vessels. This leads to loss of large amounts of blood and body fluids with widespread ischaemia. The ischaemic tissue releases toxic waste that may produce damage to the kidneys. Removal of the damaged ischaemic tissue or affected limb may be necessary. Patients may also require renal dialysis to avoid kidney damage.

Late complications

Mal-union

Mal-union refers to the union of bone fragments into an imperfect position. There is generally slight deformity in the shape of the bone following remodelling. Mal-union is important where the mal-alignment of the bone leads to shortening of the bone after fracture healing. In this case the bone fragments tend to heal with a slight overlap, and so the limb becomes shorter. In children this anomaly may remodel itself over the growing period, but in adults corrective osteotomy may be necessary, i.e. removing bone from the adjacent limb to correct the disproportion. Growth in children's bones may also be interrupted as a result of damage to the epiphyseal plates.

Post-traumatic ossification

This condition is also known as traumatic myositis ossificans. This develops as a result of repeated injury to a muscle, or a single severe injury, particularly when the injury is accompanied by extensive haemorrhage. It is thought that in damaging the muscle, osteoblasts are torn from the bone and become dislodged in the damaged muscle, which results in the local conversion of muscle into bone. Radiologically, the tissue area around the site of the fracture appears heavily calcified. This condition can be avoided by immobilizing the limb to prevent further damage and bleeding of the soft tissues around the fracture.

Osteoarthritis
See p. 264.

Failure of internal fixation

Places or pins may become loosened or dislodged due to post-operative trauma, bone disease or in some cases bone remodelling. This will cause the bone to become unstable and will require follow-up surgery.

Psychological problems

Coming to terms with long periods in bed on traction may be a problem for the patient. Road traffic accidents are producing more and more serious injuries with resultant long-term hospitalization of the patient.

A large proportion of these patients are young and their reactions to the injuries range from resentment to quiet stoicism.

PATHOLOGICAL FRACTURES

This must be treated as a separate type of fracture. Pathological fractures occur in bones where there is already underlying disease. The bone often breaks from trivial violence, or even spontaneously. The underlying disease may be localized to the bone or widespread affecting the whole skeleton. Metastases are the commonest underlying cause for pathological fractures.

Localized diseases of the bone that may also cause fractures include infections and benign and malignant tumours. General bone disorders include: congenital disorders (osteogenesis imperfecta), diffuse rarefaction of bone (senile osteoporosis) and disseminated tumours (myeloma).

Treatment of pathological fractures in most cases is by immobilization in plaster of paris and resting of the area. Fractures involving metastases usually involves a more radical approach with surgical reduction and fixation of the fracture site.

SPINE

Cervical spine

Injuries to the cervical spine are usually the result of road or sporting accidents, e.g. falls, and may be associated with head injuries. Often patients with cervical spine injuries are admitted unconscious, so the fracture is not immediately detected. The radiographer is one of the first people to handle the unconscious patient, so it is vital to treat the patient carefully, and with clinical supervision. Do not move the patient's neck, but undertake cautionary scout views of the cervical spine in the position that the patient presents.

The mechanism of injury to the cervical spine is generally due to excessive movement of the spine in any direction, e.g. flexion, extension, lateral flexion or vertical compression of the vertebral body. Flexion alone tends to cause wedge compression fractures of the cervical vertebral body. However the most serious injuries are caused by flexion and rotation. These injuries result in subluxation and/or dislocation of the spine. A flexion rotation force may also cause massive displacement of an intervertebral disc. This is then classed as an unstable fracture.

The cervical spine can also be injured by forced hyperextension. This may happen during RTAs or falls onto the face or forehead. This type of injury usually causes damage to the anterior longitudinal ligament rather than damage to the bony spine. However, hyperextension in the elderly, i.e. in the osteoarthritic cervical spine, may cause fracture to the atlas or axis, or damage to the spinal cord through impingement of bony fragments onto the cord.

Severe flexion forces may also crush the cancellous bone of one or more vertebral bodies. The compression tends to be towards the front of the vertebral bodies, thus giving it a wedge shape. The posterior ligaments remain intact making the fracture stable. More extreme burst fractures are caused when a vertical force is transmitted down the spinal column. The resulting comminuted compression fracture produces a very disrupted vertebral body that is usually stable.

Whiplash injuries are a combination of forced extension followed by forced flexion. This type of injury usually results in ligament damage only.

Treatment

In treating cervical spine injuries it is essential to have good cervical spine radiographs to demonstrate any cervical abnormality. Treatment depends on whether the injury is stable or unstable. Reduction of a dislocation or subluxation is carried out as soon after detection as possible. The injury may be treated by manipulation of the spine under image intensifier control or by continuous traction. This is applied through traction calipers that engage in small holes made in the perietal region of the skull (Figure 12.3).

Traction is maintained until fusion between the vertebrae takes place. This takes about three weeks. If stability does not return to the spine, then surgical fusion is usually carried out. The operation involves placing bone grafts to bridge the unstable joint. Plates or wires may be added to give greater stability. Pure subluxations are generally treated by immediate fusion (Clowards's operation). Wedge fractures and burst fractures, i.e. fractures of the vertical compression type, are immobilized in an orthopaedic collar. Stable extension injuries are also immobilized in collars.

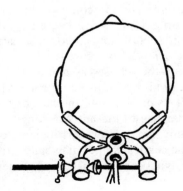

Figure 12.3   Skull calipers

Specific fractures of the cervical spine

Fractures of the atlas

The atlas is generally fractured by a vertical force acting down through the skull. The two lateral masses of the atlas are pushed aside by the downward force of the occiput. Displacement of the fragments is not severe and the spinal cord is usually undamaged. The fracture is stable and is treated by immobilizing the neck in a collar.

Fracture of the axis/odontoid process

The odontoid process usually fractures at its base. If the odontoid peg fractures, then rupture of the transverse ligament supporting the peg is rare. It tends to displace forwards in flexion injuries with little or no damage to the spinal cord. Treatment is again by skull traction using calipers followed by the fitting of a protective collar to immobilize the fracture. Occasionally anterior surgical fusion of the vertebrae is necessary.

Thoracic spine

The thoracic spine is generally very stable. Any fractures that occur are mainly caused by a vertical force acting down through the spinal column. The natural curve of the spine is predominantly one of flexion, thus most injuries are of the hyperflexion type.

Hyperflexion injuries

These tend to result in compression or burst fractures of the vertebrae. These are stable in the thoracic spine and usually only treated with rest and analgesics. However, there may be an underlying pathology in the spine that led to the fracture. Two common causes for collapse in the vertebral body are osteoporosis and metastases. These will both produce the characteristic wedge fracture. In more severe cases, paraplegia may occur.

Dislocation and fracture dislocation

The commonest displaced injury of the thoraco-lumbar spine is a fracture dislocation, usually between the levels of T10 and L2. A shearing fracture is produced that may run through the vertebral body. Paraplegia frequently results. The injury is usually caused by flexion/rotation and is a very unstable fracture. Careful management is required, with minimal movement of the patient.

Treatment is by bed rest until the fracture heals, although some cases

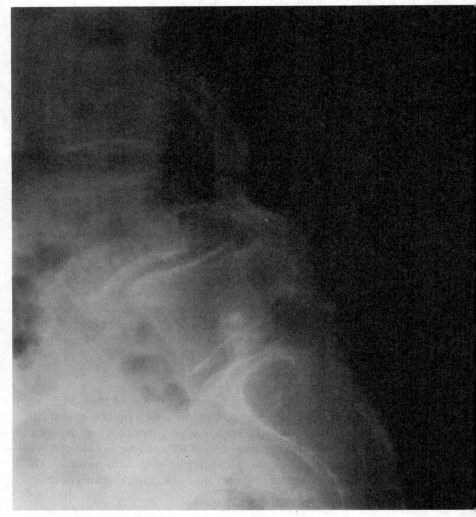

Plate 11   Spondylolisthesis

need metal plates attached to the thoracic spine to help in healing, e.g. Harrington rods. They may also be used for straightening scoliosed spines.

Lumbar region

Vertical compression

Compression and burst fractures are sometimes found in the lumbar spine as a result of blows to the head transmitted down a straight spinal column, or as a result of jumping from a height. These are essentially stable and are treated with a plaster jacket to prevent flexion and rotational movements. Vertebral fractures resulting from a fall from a height may be associated with calcaneal fractures.

The transverse processes

This type of fracture is quite common in the lumbar spine as a result of forced lateral flexion. Rarely the pars interarticularis may also fracture giving rise to a spondylolisthesis, i.e. a forward slip or subluxation of one vertebra or another. This generally happens in the L5–S1 region. Radiographically it is seen as a break in the neck of the 'scottie dog', when viewing an oblique lumbar spine radiograph (Plate 11). Treatment is by rest and analgesics.

Sacrum and coccyx

These are rare, but occasionally happen as a result of direct impact. No treatment is given unless the fragments are displaced and cause neurological or bladder problems.

Paraplegia

Fractures to the cervical spine result in complete or incomplete cord lesions:

(1) Complete cord lesions. These produce a variety of defects depending upon the level at which the lesion occurs. Any complete lesions above the level of C4 usually result in death because the respiratory muscles are paralysed. In general, complete lesions at other regions will produce anaesthesia to all stimuli, hypotonia, abolition of tendon and skin reflexes and retention of urine.
(2) Incomplete cord lesions. A number of incomplete cervical cord lesions are recognized:
    (a) The Brown-Sequard syndrome, where total loss of reflexes and

movement occurs on one side of the body with only partial loss of sensation on the opposite side.

(b) Anterior cord syndrome, where the arms become weakened but the legs are more severely paralysed.

(c) Central cord lesions, which show a combination of motor and sensory loss without any particular pattern.

Paraplegia is common in fracture dislocations of the thoraco-lumbar spine. The region affected by the cord lesion is often clinically difficult to isolate due to the region's complexity. The most common disruption to function is of bladder emptying. Emptying of the bladder is controlled by the second and third sacral segments of the spinal cord, under the ultimate control of the cerebral cortex. Loss of this control due to complete cord lesion causes loss of normal emptying. Some normal bladder emptying may take place if the reflex centres in the cord take over and control automatic bladder emptying.

SHOULDER AND UPPER ARM

Clavicle

Fractures of the clavicle are usually caused by falls onto the outstretched hand. The clavicle generally fractures at the junction of the middle and outermost thirds. If displacement occurs it is downwards and medially. This may lead to compression of the brachial plexus or axillary artery.

The fracture generally heals well with no mal-union. Treatment consists of supporting the affected side in a broad sling or a figure of eight bandage, which pulls the shoulders backwards and supports the fracture. Immobilization usually lasts for three weeks. Occasionally, surgical wiring of the fragments may be required.

Scapula

The scapula is usually fractured by direct injury. Fractures are uncommon and usually require little treatment. The scapula has been found to fracture in four specific regions, depending upon the force and direction of the blow:

(1) Neck of the scapula.
(2) Acromion process.
(3) Coracoid.
(4) Body of the scapula.

Each of the four types of fracture is treated by immobilization with a sling, although physiotherapy is also used.

Dislocation of the acromio-clavicular joint

This type of injury tends to be uncommon, but may require more active treatment than fractures to the scapula and clavicle. The dislocation usually occurs through a direct fall onto the outer prominence of the shoulder, and is commonly associated with sport. The capsule of the joint is torn and the acromion is displaced downwards from the lateral end of the clavicle, giving the characteristic joint widening seen on radiographs taken with the patient stressing the joint ('weight-bearing').

The injury is usually treated with a sling in cases of mild subluxation, although surgical treatment may be required in a severe dislocation. A screw (e.g. Bosworth screw) is driven through the clavicle into the coracoid process. However, re-subluxation of the joint may occur when the screw is removed.

Dislocation of the shoulder

This type of dislocation (Plate 12 and Figure 12.4) usually occurs through a direct fall on the arm or shoulder. It usually results in an anterior (sub-coracoid) dislocation, but may more rarely be posterior or inferior. This may lead to damage of the axillary nerve or the brachial plexus. It is therefore essential that the radiographer produces a true lateral projection of the shoulder.

The dislocation must be reduced as soon after the injury is detected as possible. A number of methods are used under local or general anaesthetic. Post-reduction radiographs must be taken to show adequate reduction of the shoulder dislocation and to ensure that no fractures have been produced due to manipulation of the shoulder. The arm is usually left in a sling for three weeks. Follow-up physiotherapy is carried out to ensure full shoulder movement is retained.

Recurrent dislocation of the shoulder

In a non-recurrent or 'routine' anterior dislocation, there is usually a tear to the joint capsule when the fracture is reduced. In recurrent or traumatic dislocations, the joint capsule is stripped from the anterior glenoid cavity margin and the articular surface of the humeral head is dented postero-laterally (Bankart lesion). On AP shoulder radiographs the head of the humerus becomes very square-shaped.

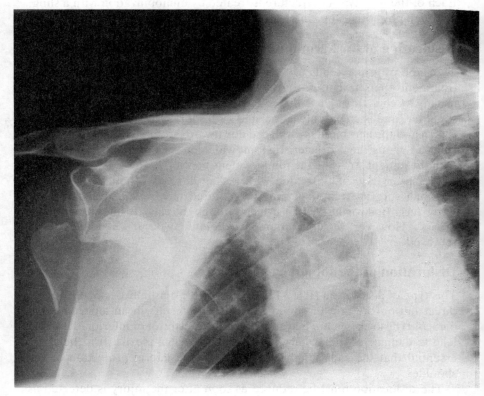

Plate 12   Fracture/dislocation of the shoulder

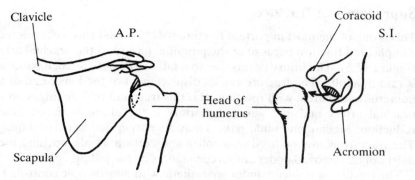

Figure 12.4 Anterior dislocation of the shoulder joint

Surgery is required to repair damage to the joint capsule, e.g. the Bankart procedure, in which the joint capsule is re-attached to the front of the glenoid.

Humerus

Neck

Fracture of the upper part of the shaft, e.g. the surgical neck, is common in the elderly, resulting from a direct fall onto the shoulder. Displacement is common, causing the head of the humerus to tilt so that the shaft of the humerus appears to either adduct or abduct. The fracture may be comminuted and impacted. The patient may complain of a stiff shoulder. Clinical examination is often tentative, and the doctor may rely on good radiographs to provide a starting point for clinical evaluation.

Treatment usually involves placing the arm in a sling with repeated physiotherapy to encourage movement. Surgical reduction and internal fixation are occasionally required. If the injury is complicated by a dislocated shoulder, then the dislocation is treated before the fracture.

In children, a slipping of the capital epiphysis from the head of the humerus is the equivalent to a fracture of the neck of the humerus. This type of injury requires reduction under anaesthesia.

Shaft

The shaft of the humerus usually fractures at its middle third, either by twisting (spiral fracture) or direct force (transverse). Pathological fractures may occur from metastatic deposits in the upper half of the humerus. Treatment is by immobilization in a collar and cuff or an upper arm plaster. Complications may involve radial nerve damage, which could give rise to wrist drop.

Supracondylar fractures

This is one of the most important fractures of childhood and is considered a complicated fracture because of the potential hazard to the brachial artery (Figure 12.5). The injury occurs due to a fall on the outstretched hand and is rare in adults. The fracture causes displacement of the lower end of the humerus backwards, with rotation. It is this fragment that impinges on the brachial artery and may sever the artery if the elbow is flexed before reduction. Median and ulnar palsies may also occur due to nerve damage. The fracture is immobilized in a collar and cuff on admission, and these must not be removed under any circumstances by the radiographer.

The fracture is reduced under anaesthetic with fluoroscopic control. The humeral fragment is rotated forward and downwards. Once reduced, follow-up radiographs are essential.

Post-operatively, the circulation is observed for twenty-four hours. Careful attention is paid to the fingers. If pain is felt in the forearm in passive extension of the fingers, then ischaemia may be developing in the muscles of the forearm. This may require exploration and grafting of the brachial artery. If the fracture remains unstable, then Kurschner wires must be driven through the fragment into the base of the fractured bone end. These are left in place for about three weeks.

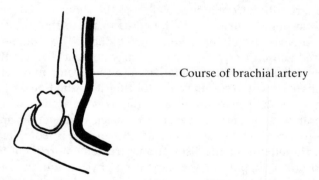

Course of brachial artery

Figure 12.5   Supracondylar fracture of the humerus

ELBOW AND FOREARM

Dislocation of the elbow

This is commonly produced by a fall on the outstretched arm. The dislocation is usually posterior, i.e. the radius and ulna are displaced posteriorly in relation to the humerus. Fractures to the elbow and damage to the median nerve or brachial artery may complicate the dislocation. Treatment consists of manipulation and reduction with or without anaesthesia and immobilization in a sling, followed up with physiotherapy. If fractures are present then open reduction is carried out with internal fixation. In extreme cases, the head of the radius may be removed and replaced with a prosthesis. Myositis ossificans may also complicate healing of fracture dislocation of the elbow.

Radial head

Fracture of the head of radius is common in young adults as a result of a fall on the outstretched arm, the force being transmitted up the arm, driving the radial head against the capitellum. Commonly the fracture is only seen on radiographs as a crack running down the head of the radius.

Elbow in children

Fractures in children usually result in disruption of the epicondyles. The fracture may displace the lateral or medial epicondyles, or the radial head may dislocate, as when the child's arm is pulled sharply.

Radius and ulna

These are caused by direct violence. A displaced fracture of the midshaft of either bone can only occur if either the radial head subluxates with an ulna fracture (Monteggia fracture) or the lower end of the ulna subluxates with a fracture of the radius (Galeazzi fracture). The fracture of both bones together is more common. Treatment is usually by open surgical reduction and fixation. Following fixation the arm is left in plaster for four to six weeks. It is essential to show good alignment to allow pronation and supination.

WRIST AND HAND

Lower end of radius

Colles fracture

The Colles fracture, first described by Abraham Colles in 1814, has come to be described as a fracture within 2.5 cm of the distal end of radius with posterior displacement and radial deviation of the distal fragment. The fracture is common in adults and may involve the distal radio-ulnar joint. The fracture presents as the characteristic 'dinner fork' deformity.

If the fracture is undisplaced, reduction may not be required. One way of assessing the need for reduction is to draw a line between the two lips of the articular surface of the radius on the lateral radiograph.

If the line is at right angles relative to the line of the radial shaft then reduction is not necessary. Any backward tilt of this line indicates a need for reduction. This is carried out under anaesthetic with the arm supported in a dorsal plaster or back slab using a sling. The plaster is usually removed after six weeks. The fragment may need plating in some extreme cases, e.g. with comminution. Occasionally median nerve compression complicates the fracture. In children the Colles fracture is equivalent to slipped lower radial epiphysis.

Smith's fracture

This is a fracture of the lower end of the radius with forward angulation of the fragment, i.e. the reverse of the Colles fracture. The fracture is generally caused by forced pronation. The fracture may be treated by immobilizing the arm in supination with a full arm plaster.

Scaphoid

Fractures of the scaphoid are frequent in adults. The most common cause is a fall onto the outstretched hand. The fracture line usually runs transversely through the middle of the scaphoid with very little displacement. This can result in avascular necrosis of the scaphoid because the proximal fragment may be deprived of its blood supply. The fracture is often small. If a fracture is clinically suspected but is not visible on radiographs, then the wrist is plastered and further radiographs obtained ten days later. Callus may then be seen around the area of the fracture. The plaster extends from the knuckles to the mid forearm, and remains in place until union is complete, usually six weeks. If no union occurs then the fracture may be treated by screw fixation or excision of any necrotic fragments induced by ischaemia.

Bennett's fracture (Plate 13)

The most common fracture injury to the thumb is Bennett's fracture. This is a fracture dislocation of the carpo-metacarpal joint of the thumb. It is a difficult fracture to reduce and may require open surgical fixation. Usually the fracture is treated by extending the thumb and then applying a plaster of paris. The thumb remains in plaster for about six weeks. As with all injuries to the wrist and hand, particularly those involving joints, osteoarthritis may develop as a later complication of the fracture.

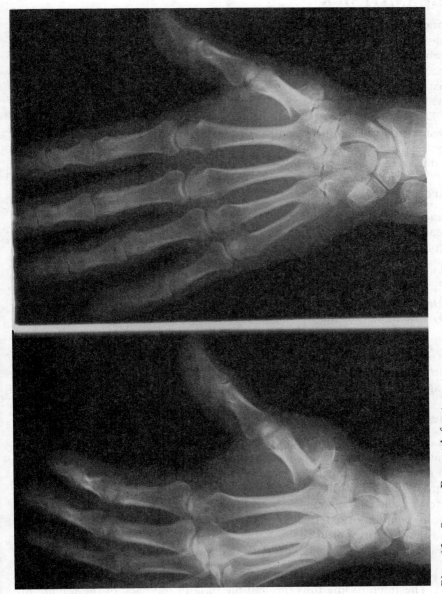

Plate 13   Severe Bennett's fracture

HIP AND FEMUR

Fractures to the pelvis occur most commonly as a result of severe trauma, e.g. road accidents and industrial accidents. The pelvis is an inherently stable ring structure. Fractures that do not enter the ring, e.g. fractures of the pubic rami, are stable and cause little damage. Unstable fractures cause disruption to the ring in two or more places and may produce disruption to the bladder, urethra and rectum.

Dislocations of the pelvis and hip also happen due to road accidents. Dislocation of the hip is usually posterior, which may result in damage to the sciatic nerve. The dislocation is usually treated by skin traction. This reduces the dislocation and allows healing of the joint capsule.

Acetabulum

Fractures of the acetabulum are associated with subluxation of the femoral head. Fractures of the acetabulum have been classed by Judet into four types:

(1) Transverse fractures of the acetabulum.
(2) Fracture of the ilio-pubic column.
(3) Fracture of the posterior rim of the acetabulum.
(4) Fracture of the ilio-ischial column.

It is essential to take oblique radiographs (Judet's views) to confirm which region is fractured. Treatment of the fractures involves traction to reduce the dislocation and may be followed by an open reduction of the fracture fragments.

Neck of the femur

Fractures of the femoral neck are very common in the elderly and are classed as pathological because there is generally underlying osteoporosis. In most cases the fracture is as a result of a rotational force acting on the femur. Generally, the shaft fragment is displaced upwards and rotated laterally, or the fragments are impacted. The fracture usually presents with the patient's foot externally rotated to as much as 90 degrees. The limb may also be foreshortened.

Fractures of the proximal part of the femur are divided into two types:

(1) Intratrochanteric. This type of fracture is found in younger patients. The fracture line runs through the base of the neck of the femur. In young patients, the limb is left on traction until union takes place. In older patients, internal fixation is carried out. A sliding type of pin and

plate is used. The dynamic hip screw allows the nail portion of the pin and plate to move, so that on weight-bearing the fracture begins to compact making the limb more stable.

(2) Intracapsular fractures. Here, the fracture line runs through the femoral neck. This is a more complicated fracture because blood supply to the head of the femur is disrupted. This may result in ischaemic necrosis of the femoral head. The fracture therefore has a poor prognosis and must be treated by immediate internal fixation. This is by a simple nail through the femoral neck, or replacement with a total hip prosthesis which requires excision of the head of femur.

Femoral shaft

These occur in all age groups and may be compound. They are usually a result of direct force, e.g. motorcycle accidents, and are treated by:

(1) Cast brace. This uses a full leg plaster or frame that is hinged at the knee and is attached at the ankle and hip. This provides rigid support of the fracture and may reduce the time required for skeletal traction. This allows weight-bearing sooner than simple traction does.

(2) Traction. Some patients may be given immediate skeletal traction, with a pin (e.g. Steinmann) placed through the calcaneum or tibia. This allows slight movement of the fracture site (Figure 12.6).

(3) Kuntscher intramedullary nail. This is used for pathological fractures and for fractures with non-union. The 'K' nail is driven through the top of the femur, across the fracture site and sits just above the knee. As it is important that the nail does not pass into the knee, fluoroscopic control is used. Union of the fracture takes about sixteen weeks, but may result in some limb shortening.

(4) The fracture may be plated and immobilized using a plaster cast brace.

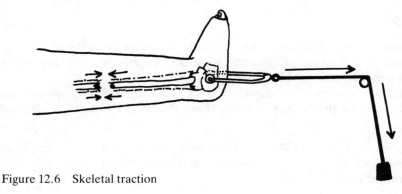

Figure 12.6   Skeletal traction

KNEE

Patella

Fractures of the patella are caused by direct violence to the knee. Transverse and comminuted fractures are common. The quadriceps muscle tends to pull the fragments apart. The fracture is usually treated by placing the knee in a full-length leg plaster, or by open internal fixation.

Upper tibia

These are caused by a direct blow to the knee and may be complicated by extending up through the tibial plateau into the knee joint capsule. This injury may also involve tears of the ligaments (lateral, medial and cruciate) and the menisci of the knee. The injury is immobilized on traction and may require internal fixation to hold the fragments in place. Complications include osteoarthritis.

Tibial shaft

Fractures of the shaft tend to be spiral or transverse and both fractures require reduction. Spiral fractures require skeletal traction. Steinmann pins may be inserted above and below the fracture, through the tibial shaft, to hold the fracture in good alignment to enable union to take place. A cast brace may also be used. Internal fixation of the fracture using plates carries the risk of osteomyelitis, particularly if there is a compound fracture present.

ANKLE AND FOOT

Ankle

Fractures to the ankle are very common. There are many variations of fractures and fracture dislocations, and they are grouped together under the general title of 'Pott's fractures'.

Fractures of the ankle are classified by the way the fracture happened and the stability of the fractured ankle. Thus the 'Pott's fracture' is divided into:

(1) Inversion injuries. This produces an avulsion fracture with displacement of the tip of the lateral malleolus. The fracture is called unimalleolar.

(2) Inversion and external rotation injuries.
(3) Eversion and external rotation injuries. These are the most complicated of the Pott's fractures, causing spiral fractures of the fibula, bimalleolar fractures and 'trimalleolar' fractures, where an anterior fragment of the tibial articular surface is displaced posteriorly. This gives the impression of three malleoli.
(4) Vertical compression fracture. This is due to a fall on the ankle and foot, causing the talus to be forced up into the tibia. This fracture is associated with fractures of the calcaneum.

Treatment

(1) Unimalleolar injuries. These fractures are quite stable and may be immobilized in plaster for satisfactory union. An above-knee plaster is used to prevent rotation of the limb.
(2) Bimalleolar injuries. These are unstable and are usually treated by internal fixation of the fragments, usually by plating the fibula.
(3) Trimalleolar injuries. These are also unstable and require internal fixations (Figure 12.7).

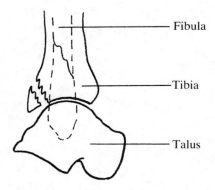

Figure 12.7 Trimalleolar fracture in lateral position

Calcaneum

These are caused by falls from a height onto the heels. They are frequently bilateral, and may be associated with fractures of the spine. The fractures tend to run through the body of the calcaneum and may disrupt the subtalar joint. These fractures are treated by immobilization and may require Steinmann pins to support the calcaneum and promote union.

Metatarsals and toes

March fracture

This is a common transverse fracture of the neck of the second metatarsal and is a typical stress fracture.

Fifth metatarsal

This is another common fracture and is caused by an inversion strain of the foot and may be associated with fractures of the ankle.

13
DISEASES OF THE ENDOCRINE SYSTEM

The endocrine glands secrete hormones directly into the bloodstream. The hormones act on target organs and help regulate body function.

THE PITUITARY GLAND

The pituitary gland (Figure 13.1) lies in the pituitary fossa of the sphenoid bone. The gland is continuous with the hypothalamus which lies above the pituitary gland. The hypothalamus is connected via the infundibulum which contains an extensive collection of vessels. The gland is subdivided into an anterior and posterior portion.

The anterior portion is called the adenohypophysis and is further subdivided into the pars distalis and pars tuberalis which surrounds the infundibular stem and is traversed by a large number of blood vessels. The adenohypophysis contains a number of cell types that are classified by the type of hormone they secrete, e.g. the corticotrophs secrete adenocorticotrophic hormone (ACTH).

The posterior lobe or pars nervosa is connected by nerve tracts to the hypothalamus.

The two sections are divided by a section of tissue called the pars intermedia. This is a very indeterminate area that is much more obvious in other animals.

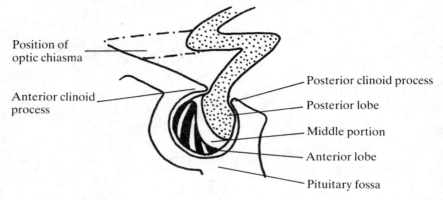

Position of optic chiasma

Anterior clinoid process

Posterior clinoid process

Posterior lobe

Middle portion

Anterior lobe

Pituitary fossa

Figure 13.1 Pituitary gland

Pituitary hormones

Anterior lobe

Thyroid-stimulating hormone (TSH or thyrotrophin)

This only affects the thyroid gland. TSH stimulates the thyroid gland to synthesize and release thyroid hormones. Release of TSH is stimulated by thyrotrophin-releasing hormone (TRH) which is secreted by the hypothalamus. Levels of thyroid hormones in the bloodstream control the release of TSH.

Follicle-stimulating hormone (FSH)

This stimulates the development of the follicle in the ovary. In the male FSH stimulates the germinal epithelium of the testicular tubules to produce sperm (spermatogenesis).

Luteinizing hormone (LH) or interstitial cell-stimulating hormone

In the female LH induces ovulation, promotes the development of the follicle and formation of the corpus luteum. In males LH stimulates interstitial (Leydig) cells to release androgens, e.g. testosterone. Release of LH and FSH is controlled by luteinizing or follicle-stimulating hormone releasing hormone (LH or FSH-RH) which is secreted to the anterior lobe of the pituitary gland by the hypothalamus.

Growth hormone (GH or somatotrophin)

This promotes growth. Release of GH is controlled by somatostatin. This is released from the hypothalamus and has an inhibitory effect on the release of GH.

Adrenocorticotrophin (ACTH)

ACTH stimulates the formation and release of the corticosteroids by the adrenal cortex. ACTH release is controlled by corticotrophin releasing factor (CRF).

Prolactin

This is essential for normal lactation. Prolactin is also necessary for fertility. Prolactin release is controlled by an inhibiting hormone secreted by the hypothalamus.

With most anterior pituitary hormones there is a feedback system operating between the level of hormone in the bloodstream secreted by the target organ and the amount of stimulating hormone released by the pituitary gland.

Posterior lobe

Two structurally similar hormones are released from the pars nervosa:

(1) Vasopressin (antidiuretic hormone or ADH). This has the effect of making the urine more concentrated by increasing the amount of water reabsorbed by the distal tubule of the renal nephron. Release of ADH is controlled by osmoreceptors situated in the anterior hypothalamus. These are stimulated by changes in the concentration of the plasma.
(2) Oxytocin. This stimulates the release of milk from the breast and causes contraction of the uterus at childbirth. Release of oxytocin is by direct neural stimulation of the pituitary gland, e.g. the child suckling stimulates oxytocin release.

ADH and oxytocin are synthesized in the hypothalamus. They are bound to the protein neurophysin and pass along the nerve tracts that connect the hypothalamus to the posterior pituitary. The hormones become concentrated in the pituitary gland before being released into the bloodstream.

Hypopituitarism

Hypopituitarism is a general term used to describe under-secretion of one or more of the pituitary hormones. The loss of hormone secretion is never uniform and a wide range of conditions are found. Disruption of the hypothalamus may produce similar effects to those found with damage to the pituitary gland.

Causes

(1) Pituitary tumours (see p. 300).
(2) Other tumours. Hypothalamic tumours, e.g. craniopharyngioma may compress or destroy the pituitary gland.
(3) Surgery and radiotherapy may be used to control pituitary tumours. This may lead to complete destruction of the gland.
(4) Infarction. Infarction of the blood supply following severe trauma to the pituitary gland, or in the presence of a tumour will cause complete loss of function of the anterior pituitary. This may also occur after severe post partum bleeding (Sheehan's syndrome).

Effects

The effects produced by hypopituitarism depend upon the age of the patient:

(1) GH deficiency. This has little effect in adults. In children impairment to GH secretion leads to small stature. This is checked by taking radiographs of the dominant hand and wrist and comparing the radiographs to a standard atlas. A discrepancy in bone age indicates a disruption to growth, e.g. a lack of GH (uncommon). Erosion of the pituitary fossa may also be demonstrated. Small stature is also seen in hypothyroidism and with disruption to the secretion of gonadotrophins.
(2) Prolactin deficiency. This produces failure of lactation. This is associated with Sheehan's syndrome.
(3) LH, FSH deficiency. Under-secretion of the gonadotrophins in children causes delayed puberty and disruption to growth. In adults lack of gonadotrophins causes an absence of body hair, osteoporosis, development of fine wrinkled skin and changes in stature. Impotence and amenorrhoea may also develop.
(4) TSH deficiency produces secondary hypothyroidism (see p. 304).

Diagnosis

Measurement of blood hormone levels is carried out. Radiography is useful in the search for pituitary tumours and in detection of bone age.

Treatment

Treatment is by hormone replacement therapy. If a tumour is present then surgical removal is carried out. Any loss of pituitary gland function is counteracted with hormone replacement therapy.

Posterior lobe

Under-secretion of ADH is the only recognized hormonal disruption of the posterior portion of the pituitary gland. Deficiency of oxytocin produces no effect.

Diabetes insipidus

This condition is caused by a deficiency in the secretion of ADH. This may be due to:

(1) Tumours of the hypothalamus.
(2) Head injuries.
(3) Surgery. Surgery to the pituitary gland area often results in diabetes insipidus. This is usually transient.

Deficiency of ADH causes the production of large amounts of dilute urine (polyuria). Treatment is by replacement of the ADH in the form of nasal sprays and intramuscular or intravenous injections.

Hyperpituitarism

Anterior lobe

Over-secretion of GH, ACTH and prolactin are commonest.

GH

Functioning pituitary tumours, e.g. adenoma, cause over-production of GH. In children and before fusion of the epiphyses over-secretion of GH causes a uniform increase of size—gigantism. Over-secretion of GH after epiphyseal fusion produces acromegaly with widespread effects. The hands and jaw become enlarged, the features become heavy and prominent, there is an increase in the thickness of subcutaneous tissue. Hypertension and diabetes mellitus may also result. Various methods are used to detect abnormalities of GH:

(1) Changes in the appearance of the patient become self-evident.
(2) Measurement of blood GH levels are carried out.
(3) Radiography of the pituitary gland may show bony erosion of the floor of the pituitary fossa. This is due to the presence of a tumour expanding and destroying the pituitary fossa.
(4) CT is also used to demonstrate functioning tumours.
(5) Soft tissue radiographs of the heel may be carried out to show an increase in the thickness of the subcutaneous tissue.

Destruction of the pituitary gland may be carried out through surgery or radiotherapy to obliterate adenomas.

Prolactin

Over-secretion of prolactin is usually due to the presence of an adenoma. This produces disruption to the menstrual cycle and infertility in women.

ACTH

Over-secretion of ACTH usually results in Cushing's syndrome (see p. 311).

Posterior lobe

Syndrome of inappropriate ADH secretion (SIADH)

This is a secondary disease and is always associated with an underlying condition. The condition may be caused by head injuries, ADH-secreting tumours, brain tumours and by carcinoma of the bronchus. The condition produces water retention. In severe cases water retention may result in brain oedema and loss of consciousness. The condition is treated by restricting fluid intake and treating the underlying disease.

Tumours

Tumours of the pituitary gland are classified as adenomas. Ademonas are benign tumours of glandular origin and are subdivided into micro- and macroadenomas. Adenomas larger than 10 mm in diameter are categorized as macroadenomas. Adenomas are further classified by the effect they produce upon hormone secretion. A distinction is made between hyper-secreting and hypo-secreting tumours. Adenomas do not occur in the posterior lobe.

Common hyper-secreting tumours are the prolactin-producing microadenomas that produce infertility in women. ACTH-producing microadenomas commonly cause Cushing's syndrome. GH-producing tumours are also usually microadenomas.

Hypo-secreting tumours do not occur as frequently as hyper-secreting tumours. Their size and growth varies widely and they may first show their presence through compression of surrounding structures as they grow out of the sella. Extrasellar extension may occur upwards, causing blockage of the foramen of Monro and compression of the optic chiasma, laterally into the cavernous sinus, causing disruption of III, IV, V and VI cranial nerves, or forwards into the frontal lobe, causing psychiatric problems.

Diagnosis

Radiographs of the sella turcica show a variety of changes. Intrasellar adenomas may cause erosion of the floor of the sella producing a classical double line across the floor when radiographs are taken in the lateral position. This may be mimicked with poor radiographs that are not taken in the true lateral position. Erosion and destruction of the clinoids may also be seen. High definition CT scanning of the pituitary fossa is usually carried out with contrast media to demonstrate microadenomas.

Treatment

Surgery

This is commonly used for treating tumours of the pituitary gland. The pituitary fossa is approached by the trans-sphenoidal approach. A small incision is made to the side of the nasal septum and this is continued into the sphenoidal sinus. This is carried out under radiographic control. An operating microscope aids in removal of all parts of the tumour. This technique will also improve any disruption caused to sight and will preserve pituitary function with little disruption to the gland. Post-operative hormone therapy is given to promote normal endocrine function. Radiotherapy may be given post-operatively to eradicate any residual active tissue.

THE THYROID GLAND

The thyroid (Figure 13.2) consists of two lateral lobes joined by an isthmus of tissue and is held closely to the trachea. The gland is formed from a number of lobules. Each lobule contains a collection of follicles lined by microvilli. Within the follicles lie the parafollicular cells or C cells which secrete calcitonin.

Iodine is essential for normal cell metabolism. The thyroid gland removes iodine from the bloodstream in the form of iodide. Once in the follicles this is combined with a protein complex to form mono- and di-iodotyrosine. It is by combination of these compounds that the thyroid hormones thyroxine (T4) and tri-iodothyronine (T3) are formed.

The hormones are stored in a colloid within the follicles of the gland and are released directly into the bloodstream. Most of the hormone released into the blood is in the form of T4. T3 is the most active form.

The main affect of thyroid hormones is in regulating cell metabolism. Lack of thyroid hormones causes a decrease in cell metabolism.

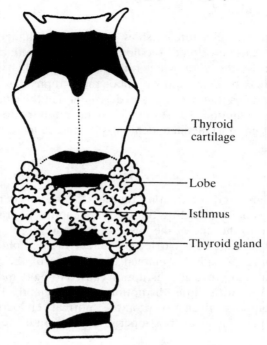

Figure 13.2   Position of the thyroid gland

The thyroid is controlled by TSH. This is released by the anterior pituitary gland. Release of TSH is regulated by the level of thyroid hormones in the blood plasma. This is a biofeedback mechanism.

Thyroid gland function is monitored by measuring the uptake and release of radioactive iodine (131I).

Inflammatory disease

Hashimoto's disease

This occurs mainly in adults and is sometimes described as autoimmune thyroiditis. An autoimmune reaction is thought to take place resulting in destruction of the thyroid. This is supported by the presence of thyroid autoantibodies in the blood of affected patients. The condition presents with swollen thyroid gland (goitre). The gland is sometimes painful to the touch. The patient usually has lowered levels of T3 and T4 in the bloodstream. Radioisotope uptake is often normal. The gland appears infiltrated by lymphatic tissue with disruption of the follicles.

The condition has been connected with other autoimmune diseases, e.g. pernicious anaemia, because antibodies to both intrinsic factor and the thyroid gland have been found in the gastric juice. The condition may be treated by giving maintenance doses of thyroxine to help promote levels of thyroid hormones.

Goitre

A goitre is any enlargement of part or all of the thyroid gland.

Simple

This is a diffuse regular enlargement of the thyroid gland, and is of two types according to cause:

(1) Iodine deficiency. This is usually due to a lack of dietary iodine. The intake of iodine per day should be approximately 150 g per day. If the level falls to approximately 50 g per day a compensatory goitre develops in an effort to extract more iodine from the diet. This is sometimes called an endemic or colloid goitre. The condition is treated by addition of iodine to the diet.
(2) No known cause. In some cases the thyroid gland enlarges with no apparent reason. Goitre is common in young women and usually produces no symptoms. It is probably associated with growth and requires no treatment. This is called a sporadic goitre. In cases of severe enlargement of the gland removal of part of it may be required.

Toxic (Graves' disease, exophthalmic goitre)

Toxic goitre is more common in women. The condition usually occurs between the ages 20–40. The patient shows a diffuse enlargement of the thyroid. This condition is one of the commonest causes of hyperthyroidism. This condition is described in the next section.

Hyperthyroidism

The patient may present with a wide variety of symptoms. Generally the patient appears overactive, underweight, agitated and has a high resting pulse rate. The patient may also have the characteristic prominent eyes (exophthalmos). Exophthalmos is due to an increase in the bulk of the muscles and other tissues around the eye. This causes the eye to bulge forwards. The upper eyelid may also become retracted causing a delay in eyelid movement (lid-lag).

In Graves' disease there is a thyroid antibody (thyroid-stimulating immunoglobulin (TSI)) present in the blood that acts on the TSH receptor site and stimulates the thyroid to over-produce T4 and T3. The gland is inflamed and shows infiltration of lymphoid tissue as with Hashimoto's disease. Levels of T3 and T4 are used to diagnose the disease.

Treatment

(1) Drugs. Iodine is given to suppress the release of thyroid hormone. The effects of iodine are short-lived and produce no long-term effects. A group of drugs called theocarbamides may also be used to treat the condition. Carbimazole is often used. This blocks the synthesis of thyroid hormones and is given as a long-term treatment in tablet form.

(2) Radioiodine. This is given as a suspension of radioactive 131I in water. The isotope is selectively absorbed and causes destruction of areas of the gland. The long-term effects of the isotope may produce hypothyroidism. Its use and dosages are closely monitored.

(3) Surgery. Surgery usually involves removal of most of the gland. Patients are given iodine prior to the operation to reduce the levels of thyroid hormone. Surgery must be carefully carried out to preserve the parathyroid glands. Removal of parts of the gland usually return the remaining gland to normal function. The surgery may induce hypo- or hyperthyroidism in a small percentage of cases.

Prognosis

Treatment produces a variety of effects. These range from complete to partial remission. Remission from Graves' disease may be obtained with theocarbamide.

Hypothyroidism

Hypothyroidism is an under-secretion of hormones from the thyroid gland. This may occur in children or in adults. It is also known as myxoedema in adults.

Neonatal or congenital (cretinism)

This occurs in utero and is obvious at birth or in early life. The fetus relies upon production of its own supply of thyroid hormones and receives very little from the mother. Therefore, failure of the thyroid gland to develop while in utero causes a wide range of changes in the child due to failure of the tissues to develop and mature. The child has some form of brain damage, very coarse facial features, prominent tongue and abdominal problems, including umbilical hernia. Coarse, disrupted epiphyses are demonstrated on radiographs of the bones.

Adult

This occurs in all age groups and is more common in females.

Causes

(1) Absence of dietary iodine.
(2) Surgery. Removal of portions of the thyroid in treating hyperthyroidism may cause hypothyroidism.
(3) Therapeutic irradiation of the thyroid.
(4) Hashimoto's disease. Thyroid antibodies are found in many patients with hypothyroidism.

Symptoms

(1) Myxoedema. Particles of protein-rich material are found in the thyroid.
(2) Metabolism is slowed. The patient complains of lethargy, slow mental ability and of feeling cold. Bradycardia, coarse skin and loss of hair are also common.

Treatment

Hypothyroidism may be treated by giving thyroxine in tablet form.

Tumours

Benign

Adenoma of the thyroid gland is a common benign tumour of the gland. Some types of active adenomas ('hot') may produce hyperthyroidism due to the presence of thyroid antibodies that stimulate the thyroid gland to produce hormones. Non-active adenomas ('cold') usually cause no physiological effects. The distinction between hot and cold is made by radioisotope scans of the thyroid.

Malignant

This accounts for only approximately 1 per cent of all carcinomas. The incidence is higher in people who have had a previous goitre.

Types

(1) Papillary. This occurs at any age. The primary tumour may have single or multiple elements in the thyroid. Spread to both lobes of the gland is

common. Spread to local lympth nodes, e.g. cervical, is common. Spread of metastases by the blood is only a late complication of the tumour. Prognosis is good for this type of tumour.

(2) Follicular. This type occurs later in life. Spread to lymph nodes is not as common as with papillary carcinomas. A more aggressive form occurs in the elderly.

(3) Anaplastic. This is the least common carcinoma of the thyroid. It is a highly malignant tumour with a poor prognosis that most frequently occurs in the elderly. Spread to the lymphatics and blood is common.

(4) Medullar. This is a rare form of thyroid tumour that affects the parafollicular cells and stimulates increased release of calcitonin.

Diagnosis

(1) Goitre is usually apparent.
(2) Ultrasound may show the presence of cysts and masses.
(3) Uptake of 131I may show a lesion.
(4) History of dietary deficiency of iodine, a history of goitre and curative irradiation to the thyroid gland may all prompt tumour formation.

Treatment

Carcinoma is usually treated by removal of the complete affected node. In some cases, e.g. papillary tumour, this may be followed by further surgery to the other lobe. Removal of local lymph nodes may also be carried out to prevent spread. Preservation of the parathyroids is always attempted. Surgery may be followed by theraputic doses of 131I to destroy any residual cancer cells. Papillary tumours do not respond well to treatment of 131I. Anaplastic tumours are very difficult to treat. Treatment tends to be palliative.

Treatment of thyroid tumours produces complications, including hypothyroidism, recurrent nerve damage and loss of parathyroid function. Replacement therapy is frequently required together with routine checks of general health.

THE PARATHYROIDS

There are four parathyroid glands (Figure 13.3) lying within the body of the thyroid gland. Two lie in the superior portion of the thyroid lobes and two lie inferiorly. The position of the glands is variable.

The parathyroids secrete parathyroid hormone (PTH). PTH has a number of effects:

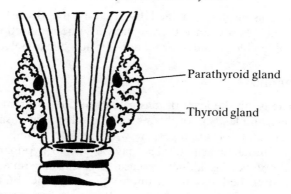

Parathyroid gland

Thyroid gland

Figure 13.3   Posterior view of the thyroid gland showing the position of the parathyroid glands

(1) It promotes osteoclast activity to liberate calcium and phosphates.
(2) It acts on the kidney tubules and reduces the reabsorption of phosphate and increases the reabsorption of calcium.

The overall effect is to raise plasma calcium and lower plasma phosphates. The secretion of PTH is controlled by a feedback system. High calcium ion concentration in the plasma inhibits PTH, low calcium ion concentration prompts PTH release. Calcium and phosphate are essential for normal cell metabolism.

Lying among the follicular cells of the thyroid are the parafollicular or C cells which secrete the hormone calcitonin. This is thought to oppose the effect of PTH and reduce osteoclast activity.

Approximately half the calcium is absorbed by the gut under a system that depends upon vitamin D for its function. Loss of calcium is via the gut and the urine. Resorption by the kidney tubules under the influence of PTH controls release of calcium.

Hypercalcaemia

This is a raised level of plasma calcium. Calcium is important in normal muscle function. High levels of calcium most commonly cause muscle weakness, weight loss and constipation. Increased calcium also causes an increase in the output of urine. This condition may be due to:

(1) Hyperparathyroidism.
(2) Hyperthyroidism.
(3) Tumours of the thyroid.

The condition us usually rectified by treating the disease causing the hypercalcaemia. Maintenance therapy may also be required to rectify the salt balance of the blood and to avoid dehydration due to polyuria.

Hypocalcaemia

This is a decrease in the level of plasma calcium. An extreme decrease in the level of calcium leads to problems with muscle metabolism. Parathesia of the limbs may occur together with muscle cramps and tetany (uncontrolled muscle spasms). This may be due to hypoparathyroidism, vitamin D deficiency or kidney disease, e.g. chronic renal failure that causes an uncontrolled loss of calcium in the urine. The condition may be corrected by giving oral doses of calcium. In emergencies patients may be given calcium intravenously.

Hyperparathyroidism

This is subdivided into primary and secondary disease.

Primary

This is due to an excessive release of parathyroid hormone.

Causes

The condition is commonly caused by a tumour, usually a benign adenoma. These may be single or multiple. Carcinomas are uncommon. In the minority of cases (approximately 10 per cent), the condition is due to hyperplasia of the gland.

Symptoms

Elevated PTH produces a rise in the level of plasma calcium. This may produce:

(1) Calcification of blood vessels and renal calculi formation due to hypercalcaemia. Calcification of the renal substance (nephrocalcinosis) may also develop in severe cases.
(2) Polyuria.
(3) Constipation.
(4) Changes to bone.

Diagnosis

(1) Radiography. Bony changes may be noted due to raised PTH. The bony changes are subtle and usually occur as changes in the phalanges.

This may be demonstrated by macroradiography. Much finer techniques are now being developed to produce ultra-fine detail.
(2) Blood. Raised serum calcium levels and raised levels of PTH indicate hypercalcaemia. Raised calcium levels are accompanied by increased levels of phosphates.

Treatment

Primary hyperparathyroidism is a common complaint. Many patients are asymptomatic and are detected as having the condition through routine blood screening. Many cases are therefore treated conservatively.

Patients with adenoma require surgical removal of the tumour. This involves precise techniques and suitable localization of the tumour. This may be obtained by measuring the plasma concentrations around the thyroid, and may be carried out under radiographic control by introducing a fine catheter into the vessels feeding and leaving the thyroid. Blood samples are taken at routine positions around the gland.

Prognosis

Complete removal of the adenoma produces good results. Blood levels of calcium and phosphate are carried out post-operatively to monitor for recurrence of tumour. Very fine tumour tissues may be left behind.

Secondary

This is an increase of PTH due to the presence of another disease, usually renal failure, which persistently causes a lowered level of plasma calcium. The condition is detected by an increase in the level of blood phosphates and a decrease in the level of blood calcium due to the associated renal disease. Treatment is by management of the underlying disease.

Hypoparathyroidism

The condition may follow surgery to, or theraputic irradiation of, the thyroid gland with resultant damage to the parathyroid glands. It is diagnosed by finding a low level of PTH in the blood and is treated by giving calcium in tablet or liquid form.

THE ADRENAL GLANDS

The two adrenal glands (Figure 13.4) lie on the upper poles of the kidneys. Each gland is composed of an inner medulla and outer cortex. The medulla

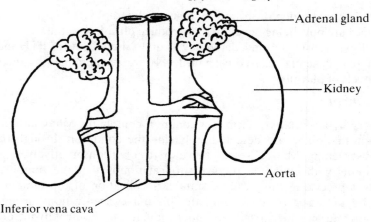

Figure 13.4   Position of the adrenal glands

contains mainly nerve tissue. The outer cortex is subdivided into three distinct layers: the outer zona glomerulosa, middle zona fasciculata and the inner zona reticularis. The two layers secrete a complex variety of hormones.

Hormones
Cortex

The adrenal cortex secretes a number of types of hormone. These are broadly subdivided into two groups:

(1) The mineralocorticoids, e.g. aldosterone. This is secreted from the zona glomerulosa. Aldosterone acts on the kidneys to produce an increase in the uptake of sodium and an increase in potassium secretion.
(2) The glucocorticoids, e.g. hydrocortisone (cortisol). Hydrocortisone is important in carbohydrate metabolism. One of its main effects is to maintain the level of glucose in the blood plasma. It does this by antagonizing the effect of insulin and promoting the conversion of proteins to glucose.
(3) The sex hormones, e.g. androgens. These are secreted by the zona reticularis.

Medulla

This secretes adrenaline and noradrenaline. These promote the overall rate of metabolism, increases heart rate and an increase in blood pressure.

Adrenal cortex

Cushing's syndrome

This is an over-secretion of the glucocorticoids, particularly hydrocortisone.

Causes

(1) Over-secretion of ACTH. This may be due to disruption of the hypothalamus or disease of the pituitary gland, e.g. microadenoma.
(2) Adrenal adenoma. This may stimulate over-secretion of hydrocortisone.
(3) Ectopic ACTH secretion. Tumours in other regions, e.g. oat cell carcinomas of the bronchus may release ACTH.

Symptoms

(1) Obesity and the typical rounded 'moon face' of the Cushing's patient.
(2) Osteoporosis.
(3) Amenorrhoea and infertility.
(4) Hypertension.
(5) Weakness and muscle wasting.

Diagnosis

Blood plasma levels will show an increase of the level of ACTH. CT scanning may show an underlying microadenoma of the pituitary gland or adenomas of the adrenal glands.

Treatment

In the case of an adrenal adenoma surgical removal of the adrenal is carried out. This is followed by corticosteroid therapy to maintain a normal level of steroid action. Pituitary microadenomas are also removed and the patients may receive short-term corticosteroid therapy following surgery.

In cases where a tumour cannot be demonstrated the aim of the treatment is to reduce the level of the corticosteroids to healthy levels. This may be achieved by removal of both the adrenals and replacing their function with permanent corticosteroid therapy. The patient must carry a card indicating that they are on steroid therapy. This is to warn medical staff who may need to treat the patient urgently.

Prognosis

Prognosis is good when the condition is treated. In cases of untreated Cushing's syndrome death may result from cardiovascular disease.

Hyperaldosteronism

Conn's syndrome (primary aldosteronism)

This is an increase in the secretion of aldosterone (a mineralocorticoid). This causes:

(1) A decrease in the level of plasma potassium (hypokalaemia) due to an increase in potassium excretion. This leads to severe muscle weakness, paralysis and parathesia.
(2) Hypertension.

This condition is commonly caused by an adenoma in the adrenal gland. Removal of the tumour usually cures the condition. The tumours are rarely malignant.

Addison's disease (chronic cortical hypofunction)

This is due to a lack of secretion of gluco- and mineralocorticoids and develops through slow destruction of the adrenal cortex. This is usually due to an autoimmune mechanism. The condition may take many years to develop and may only be obvious in the middle aged.

(1) The patient develops an increase in skin pigmentation. This is due to an over-secretion of ACTH caused by a lack of corticosteroids, which usually control ACTH secretion in a feedback mechanism.
(2) There is an increase in the loss of sodium in the urine and a rise in the level of blood potassium.
(3) Hypoglycaemia.

Diagnosis is usually through accurate estimates of the levels of ACTH and corticosteroids in the blood plasma. Treatment is through replacement therapy which is carried out using glucocorticoids, e.g. hydrocortisone. This may have to be sustained for long periods.

Acute adrenocortical hypofunction (adrenal crisis, Addisonian crisis)

This is an acute form of adrenal hypofunction and is a medical emergency. It usually occurs through a sudden lack of hydrocortisone. The patient quickly loses consciousness unless given a rapid intravenous infusion of hydrocortisone. This situation may be prompted by acute infections or omission of steroids in a patient on steroid therapy.

Over-secretion of sex hormones

The adrenals produce androgens and some oestrogen. Over-secretion of these hormones is usually caused by the presence of tumours.

Androgens

(1) Male. In adult men the condition may go undetected. In boys increased secretion produces a precocious pseudopuberty with early maturation of the penis and gonads, increase in body hair and an increase in height and body weight. Early fusion of the epiphyses may cause a stunting of height.

(2) Females. In women there is an increase in the amount of body hair with disruption to or absence of periods.

Oestrogens

(1) Male. This may promote breast development (gynaecomastia).

(2) Female. This produces irregularities of the menstrual cycle.

Adrenal medulla

Phaeochromocytoma

This is a rare tumour and usually occurs in young adults. The tumours are encapsulated and occur bilaterally in 10 per cent of all cases. In a small percentage of patients the tumour is malignant. Phaeochromocytomas may occur outside the adrenals in other areas of sympathetic nervous tissue.

The tumour causes an increase in the secretion of catecholamines, e.g. adrenaline. The condition may be associated with neurofibromatosis. The tumour also causes hypertension and a range of generalized symptoms, e.g. palpitations, episodes of sweating and weight loss due to an increase in metabolism.

Diagnosis is usually by the blood level of catecholamines. CT scanning is one of the more useful techniques of demonstrating the adrenals. High dose IVU and angiography may be carried out. Treatment is by surgical removal of the tumour.

GLOSSARY

This glossary is not exhaustive, but is designed to give an outline of general terms used when describing disease.

Abscess. Term commonly applied to a collection of pus in a tissue space, following infection. Pulmonary abscess describes an abscess in the lung.

Adenoma. A simple tumour of a solid glandular tissue.

Anaemia. A disorder in which the oxygen-carrying capacity of the blood is impaired.

Aneurysm. An abnormal dilatation of an artery.

Antibiotic. An antimicrobial agent manufactured from fungi.

Antibody. This is a product of the body's reaction to an antigen.

Antigen. This is a substance which when introduced into the body produces a specific immune response.

Ascites. An excessive build-up of fluid in the peritoneal cavity.

Atherosclerosis. A degenerative disease of the arteries.

Autosome. An autosome is one of an equal pair of chromosomes that are concerned with determination of all characteristics other than the sex of the individual. Of the forty-six chromosomes found in man, there are twenty-two pairs of autosomes and one pair of sex chromosomes.

Bacteria. Organisms that exist singly or groups and cause a variety of diseases.

BCG (Bacille Calmette-Guérin). A vaccine used for inoculation against tuberculosis.

Bence Jones protein. Specific protein found in the urine of patients with some bone marrow disorders, e.g. multiple myeloma.

Benign. Not life-threatening. Usually used to describe non-malignant tumours.

Bile. Substance secreted by the liver containing: bile pigments, cholesterol and inorganic salts.

Bleeding time. The period which blood continues to escape from a wound created in the skin without the formation of a clot (approximately 2–3 minutes).

Bronchitis. Prolonged inflammation of the bronchi.

Calcification. Deposition of calcium salts in the tissues.

Calculus. An abnormal stone-like collection of calcium salts, e.g. salivary gland calculi, renal calculi.

Callus. Area of reparative tissue surrounding the site of a fracture, formed mainly from loosely woven bone.

Cancer. Usually used to describe a malignant neoplasm.

Candida. Species of fungi. *Candida albicans* causes moniliasis ('thrush').

Cardiospasm. Generally described as spasm of the cardiac sphincter of the stomach.

Caries. Dental decay that affects the enamel. Secondary spread to the dental pulp may also occur.

Cataract. An opacity of the lens or its capsule.

Catecholamine. Term describing the neurotransmitters (adrenaline and noradrenaline) released by the adrenal medulla.

Cholangitis. Inflammation of the bile ducts.

Cholelithiasis. Gall-stones.

Chromosomes. These carry genes and transmit genetic characteristics from generation to generation. A constant number of chromosomes exist in the cells of an animal species, e.g. forty-six for the human cell. Sex chromosomes (denoted X and Y) carry the sexual characteristics of the individual. XX indicates female and XY male. Certain diseases are sex linked, i.e. usually carried on the X chromosome. These include haemophilia and Huntington's chorea.

Chronic. A disease of long duration.

Cirrhosis. A term usually applied to the liver indicating a chronic progressive disease of it, producing extensive destruction of the liver parenchyma. This results in jaundice. Cirrhosis is commonly present with alcoholism.

Coarctation. Narrowing of the lumen of a vessel or a canal. Commonly used in association with the aorta.

Colic. Severe spasmodic pain in the abdomen. Commonly described in relation to the presence of calculi in the kidney/ureter (renal colic) or in the biliary system (biliary colic).

Colitis. An inflammation of the colon.

Collapse. Commonly associated with collapse of areas of the lung. This is due to an absence of air from the lung tissue due to an obstruction to a bronchus or bronchi.

Colostomy. Creation of an artificial anus by making a direct opening through the abdomen into the colon.

Coma. Complete loss of consciousness. May be associated with uncontrolled diabetes mellitus.

Consolidation. Broadly used to describe the condition of becoming solid. Used to describe areas of the lung following extensive inflammations and infections, e.g. pneumonia.

Cyanosis. Bluish discoloration of the skin caused by improper oxygenation of the blood.

Cyst. Membranous sac containing fluid.

Demyelination. Destruction of the myelin sheathe.

Deossification. Absorption of bone.

Dialysis. Filtration through a semi-permeable membrane. Renal dialysis = filtration of the blood.

Diaphysis. Shaft of a long bone.

Diphtheria. Acute infectious disease caused by *Corynebacterium diphtheriae*.

Dislocation. Displacement of the bones of a joint. May also be used to indicate movement of an organ.

Diverticulum. Small blind-ended pouch arising from the wall of a hollow organ, e.g. bladder, bowel.

DNA. Deoxyribonucleic acid.

Dyskinesia. Impairment of involuntary movement.

Dysphagia. Difficulty in swallowing.

Dysphasia. Impairment to speech due to lesion within the central nervous system.

Dysphrasia. Impairment of speech due to disruption to mental ability.

Dysplasia. Abnormal formation of tissue.

Dyspnoea. Difficulty in breathing.

Dysuria. Pain on micturition, or difficulty in passing urine.

Eclampsia. Hypertensive toxaemia of pregnancy. Usually occurs in the latter stages of pregnancy. Exaggerated increase in blood pressure may lead to coma.

Ectopia. An abnormal position of an organ.

Effusion. Production of transudate or exudate into a serous cavity. This may occur into the pleura following infection of the lung tissue.

Embolism. Occlusion or obstruction of a blood vessel usually by a detached blood clot carried in the bloodstream.

Embolus. Any foreign material carried in the bloodstream, e.g. blood clot, metastasis, air bubble, bacteria. The embolus usually lodges in a blood vessel and causes disruption to blood flow.

Emphysema. An abnormal distension of the tissues by air.

Empyema. Pleurisy with production of pus.

Endotoxin. A toxin that is contained within the structure of a bacteria and is only liberated when the bacteria dies.

Enucleation. General term for removal of one structure from another. Also used to indicate removal of the eyeball.

Epiphysis. Distal part of a long bone, initially united with the diaphysis by cartilage.

Epistasis (stasis). Lack of movement of fluids, discharge, etc. Obstruction of the bladder causes urinary stasis.

Epitaxis. Nasal haemorrhage.

Erythema. Diffuse, patchy redness of the skin.

Fibrillation. Localized erratic contractions of muscle fibres. Usually associated with cardiac muscle.

Fistula. An abnormal channel between two, usually hollow, organs or from an organ to the skin surface.

Gangrene. Necrosis of part of the body due to lack of arterial blood supply to that part.

Gastritis. Inflammation of the gastric mucous membrane.

Gravid. Pregnant.

Haemarthrosis. Haemorrhage into a joint.

Haematemesis. The vomiting of blood.

Haematoma. A collection of extravasated blood.

Haematuria. Passage of bloodstained urine.

Haemolysis. The process of the liberation of haemoglobin from red blood cells.

Haemoptysis. The passage of blood on coughing.

Haemorrhage. The loss of blood from blood vessels.

Haemothorax. Collection of blood in the pleural cavity.

Hemiplegia. Paralysis of one side of the body.

Hiatus. An empty space or an opening. Commonly describes an hiatus hernia, where a portion of the stomach protrudes through the hiatus of the diaphragm into the chest.

Hydronephrosis. A distension of the kidney due to obstruction of the flow of urine.

Hyperplasia. An increase in the size of an organ, due to an increase in the number of cells.

Hypertension. Commonly taken to indicate increased blood pressure.

Hypertrophy. Increase in the size of a tissue due to an increase in the size of individual tissues.

Idiopathic. Spontaneous origin. With no apparent underlying cause.

Infarct. Swelling of an area of tissue due to engorgement with blood following loss of blood supply to the area of tissue.

Inflammation. The reaction of tissue following injury.

Ischaemia. Loss or restriction of blood supply.

Laparotomy. An excision through the abdominal wall. Generally taken to indicate an exploratory operation of the abdomen.

Lymphoedema. Oedema due to blockage of the lymphatic system.

Meconium. The first faecal discharge of the newborn.

Metaphysis. Distal part of the diaphysis.

Necrosis. Death of an area of tissue. May follow prolonged ischaemia.

Neural. Relating to a nerve or the nervous system. Neural tube.

Notochord. Embryonic tissue from which the vertebral spine develops.

Nystagamus. Involuntary rhythmic movements of the eye.

Oophorectomy. Removal of the ovaries.

Oophorohysterectomy. Removal of ovaries and uterus.

Paralysis. Loss of nervous function.

Plexus. Network of vessels, nerves or blood vessels.

Purulent. Marked by the formation of pus. Term connected with the formation of pus.

Salpingectomy. Excision of the uterine tube.

Salpingo-oophorectomy. Excision of the uterine tube and ovary.

Suppuration. The formation of pus.

Talipes. Club foot.

Ulcer. An erosion and loss of substance from a tissue surface.

Urticaria. An allergic reaction of the skin.

BIBLIOGRAPHY

I found the following texts useful in helping me compile this book:

Armstrong, P. and Wastie, M. L. (1983) *X-Ray Diagnosis,* Blackwell Scientific Publications, Oxford

Blandy, J. (1982) *Lecture Notes on Urology,* 3rd edition, Blackwell Scientific Publications, Oxford

Brewis, R. A. L. (1985) *Lecture Notes on Respiratory Disease,* Blackwell Scientific Publications, Oxford

Dean, M. R. E. (1975) *Basic Anatomy and Physiology for Radiographers,* Blackwell Scientific Publications, Oxford

Donnie, P. A. (ed.) (1983) *Cash's Textbook of Chest, Heart and Vascular Disorders for Physiotherapists,* Faber & Faber, London

Duckworth, T. (1984) *Lecture Notes on Orthopaedics and Fractures,* Blackwell Scientific Publications, Oxford

Ede, D. A. (1978) *An Introduction to Developmental Biology,* Blackie, London

Elias, E. and Hawkins, C. (1985) *Lecture Notes on Gastroenterology,* Blackwell Scientific Publications, Oxford

Green, J. H. (1974) *An Introduction to Human Physiology,* OUP, Oxford

International Union Against Cancer (1982) *Manual of Clinical Oncology,* Springer-Verlag, New York

Jawetz, E., Melnick, J. L. and Alelberg, E. A. (1984) *Review of Medical Microbiology,* Lange Medical Publications, Los Artos, California

Jennet, B. and Galbraith, S. (1983) *An Introduction to Neurosurgery,* Heinemann, London

Julian, D. G. (1983) *Cardiology,* Ballière Tindall, London

Macleod, J. (ed.) (1974) *Davidson's Principles and Practice of Medicine,* Churchill-Livingstone, London

Matthews, W. B. (1982) *Diseases of the Nervous System,* Blackwell Scientific Publications, Oxford

Reese, A. J. M. (1981) *The Principles of Pathology,* John Wright, Bristol

Thomson, A. D. and Cotton, R. E. (1983) *Lecture Notes on Pathology,* Blackwell Scientific Publications, Oxford

Walter, J. B. and Israel, M. S. (1979) *General Pathology,* Churchill-Livingstone, London

INDEX

abcess:
  intracranial 177-8
  liver 136
  lung 17
acetone 139
achalasia of the cardia 105-6
achondroplasia 250
acne vulgaris 194-5
acoustic neuroma 189-90
acromegaly 251
Adam-Stokes attack 72
Addison's disease 312
adenoids 11
adrenal gland anatomy 309-10
adult respiratory distress syndrome
  (ARDS) 39
aegenesis of kidney 207
Albers-Schönbergs disease: see
  osteopetrosis
Alport's syndrome 211
amylase 142
amyotrophic lateral sclerosis 182
anaemia 21, 81-4, 86, 89, 92-4, 107, 126,
  247
anencephaly 158
aneurysms 66-8
  intracranial 170-73
  kidney 223
angina-pectoris 59-60
angiofibroma 12
ankylosing spondylitis 262

antibiotics 21, 29, 130, 136, 175, 178, 250
aortic valve disease 64-5
Arnold-chiari malformation 158, 159
arterial disease:
  stenosis 73
  thrombosis 74
arterio-venous malformation 166, 167,
  173
arteriosclerosis 141
arteriovenous fistula 68
arteriovenous-malformation (AVM) 67
arthritis:
  osteo 264
  rheumatoid 183-99, 260-62
  supparative 263-4
asbestosis 33
Aschoff nodes 61
ascites 127
aspiration pneumonia 17
asthma 29 see also bronchial asthma
astroblastoma 184
astrocytoma 184
atherosclerosis 59
atrial fibrillation (AF) 71
atrial septal defect (ASD) 50-1, 70
avascular necrosis 259

Bacille-Calmette-Guérin (BCG) 23
back slab 288
bacteria 7, 53, 129, 130, 136, 140, 175,

212, 214, 215, 227, 234
Bankart lesion 283
Bence Jones protein 86, 255
Bennet's fracture 288
Berry aneurysm 67, 208
beta blocker 72
biscupid aortic valve 54
bile 128
Blalock-Taussig procedure 57
blind loop syndrome 124
blood 77-80
blood count 77-8
bone age 298
bone structure 241-2
Bosworth screw 283
bovine tuberculosis 19
bradycardia 71
brain anatomy 154-6
breast anatomy 148
breast tumours 149-52
bronchiectasis 26
    bronchography 27
    treatment 27
bronchial asthma 29-31
bronchial carcinoma 15, 29-31, 33, 39-41,
    bronchitis 42, 300
    chronic 23-4
    treatment 24
bronchodilators 29, 30, 32, 33
bronchopneumonia 16
Brown-Sequard syndrome 281-2
bullae 26

Cafe-au-lait 187
Caisson's disease 260
calculi:
    gall bladder 129-33
    renal 130, 212, 214, 220-22, 308
callus formation 271
candida albicans 99
carcinoid syndrome 124
carcinomatosis peritonei 127
cardiomyopathy 68
cardiothoracic ratio (CTR) 44, 46
cast brace 291
cataracts 141, 190-91
cavitation 21
cerebro-vascular accident (CVA) 167

cerebrospinal fluid (CSF) 156-7
cervical cancer 238-9
cervical spine injuries 277-8
Charcot joints 141, 264-5
cheilities 93
chemotherapy 41, 82, 84, 86, 95, 126,
    138, 143, 146, 147, 234, 236, 239, 255,
chest anatomy 13-14
chest drain 37
cholecystitis:
    acute 129
    chronic 130
chondroblastoma 253
chondroma 253
chondrosarcoma 253
chronic asthma 30
chronic bronchitis 9
chronic obstructive airways disease
    (COAD) 23, 25
Cimino fistulae 217
cirrhosis 136, 137
claudication 74
cleft palate 98
Cloward's operation 278
coalworker's pneumoconiosis (CWP): *see*
    pneumoconiosis
coarctation 54
Codman's triangle 252
coeliac disease 120-1
Colles fracture 287-8
condyloma acuminata 195
congenital dislocation of the hips (CDH)
    1, 257-8
congenital heart disease 49-57
Conn's syndrome 69, 225, 312
connective tissue anatomy 198
continuous ambulatory peritoneal
    dialysis (CAPD) 217, 218, 219
craniopharyngioma 187
craniostenosis 158
cretinism 304
Crohn's disease 114-17, 118, 120, 123,
    127, 212
crush syndrome 275
Cushing's syndrome 69, 219, 244, 311
cyanosis 14, 33, 55, 124
cystic fibrosis 27-9, 68
cystitis 227-9

cysts:
  bone 256, 258
  kidney 207
  liver 208
  lung 208
  pancreas 142, 208
  salivary 101

dacron 51
deep vein thrombosis (DVT) 76, 274
dermatitis 194
dermoid cyst 42
dextrocardia 50, 108
diabetes mellitus 59, 138-41, 183, 210-11
diabetes insipidus 299
dialysis 141
diamorphine 60
diaphragmatic hernia 42
diarrhoea 124, 126
diptheria 13
disease 1
dislocation:
  acromio-clavicular joint 283
  elbow 286-87
  shoulder 283-5
diverticulae:
  bowel 121
  oesophagus 106
diverticular disease 121-2
diverticulitis 121
diverticulosis 121
Down's syndrome 50, 83
duplex ureter 209
dynamic hip screw 291
dyschondroplasia 250-51
dyspnoea 15, 22

ectopic kidney 205-6
eczema 194
electrocardiogram (ECG) 47-9
emphysema 25-6
  surgical 25
empyema 42
encephalitis 177, 180
end stage kidney 211
endoscopic retrograde
  choledochopancreatography (ERCP)

130, 133, 142, 143
enucleation 191
ependymoma 185
epilepsy 177, 178, 187-8
Epstein-barr virus 147
erythrocytic sedimentation rate (ESR) 80
erythema nodosum 20, 31
Ewing's tumour 254
exophthalmos 303
extradural haemmorhage 166
exudate 42

Fallot's tetralogy 54
fat embolism 275
fibroadenoma 149
fibroma 253-4
fibrosarcoma 254
finger clubbing 13-14
fistula 119, 122, 126
fractures:
  ankle and foot 292-3
  atlas 279
  axis 279
  calcaneum 293
  categories 266-8
  children 269-70
  healing 270
  hip and femur 290-91
  humeral neck 285
  humeral shaft 285
  metatarsals 294
  patella 292
  radial head 287
  radius and ulna 287
  sacrum and coccyx 279
  scapula 282-3
  tibia 292
  wrist and hand 287-90
Frieberg's disease 259
fungi 17, 21, 137

Galaezzi fracture 287
gangrene 9, 75, 274
gastritis 111-12
German measles (rubella) 50
Ghon focus 20
gigantism 251

glaucoma 141, 191
gliomas 184-5, 192
glomerulonephritis 210
glossitis 93
gluten 120
glyceryl trinitrate 59
glycosuria 139
goitre 302, 303, 306
gonococcal urethritis 234
gout 262
grand mal 187-8
Graves' disease 303
Grawitz tumour 225-6
Guillan-Barre syndrome 184
gynaecomastia 153, 313

haemangioma 12, 137, 255
haematuria 205
haemmorhoids 75
haemodialysis 217-18
haemoglobinopathies 87-90
haemophilia A 90-91
haemophilia B 91
haemoptysis 15, 27, 40
hare lip 98
Harrington rods 279
Hashimoto's disease 302-3, 305
Heaf test 22-3
heart block 72
heart size 44-7
hemiplegia 167, 168
hepatitis A 135
hepatitis B 135, 137
herpetic stomatitis 99
hiatus hernia 42, 104-5
Hirschsprung's disease 112-13, 123
Hodgkin's disease 145-7
horseshoe kidney 205-6
human immunodeficiency virus (AIDS)
   10, 198
Huntington's chorea 181-2
hyaline membrane disease: *see*
   respiratory distress syndrome
hydrocephalus 158-61, 164
hydrocoele 235
hydronephrosis 204
hypercalcaemia 307-8
hypercalcuria 244

hyperglycaemia 138
hyperkeratosis 194
hyperparathyroidism 220-21, 246, 307,
   308-9
hyperpituitarism 299-300
hypertension 54, 68-70, 167, 224-5, 312
hyperthyroidism 244, 303, 307
hypertrophic obstructive cardiomyopathy
   (HOCM) 68
hypocalcaemia 308
hypoglycaemia 140, 312
hypoparathyroidism 309
hypopituitarism 95, 297-9
hypothyroidism 304-5

infection 7-9
inguinal hernia 123-4
insulin 140
intestines anatomy 112
intracerebral haemmorhage 167
intussusception 122, 123, 124, 127

Kaposi's sarcoma 198
Kerley B lines 63
ketoacidoaia 139
kidney anatomy 203-4
Kienbock's disease 259
Klinfelter's syndrome 240
Klippel-Feil abnormality 164
Kohler's disease 259
Kuntscher nail 291
Kveim test 31

laryngitis 13
larynx anatomy 13
Legionnaire's disease 17
leiomyoma 237
leukaemia 83-7
levodopa 181
linitis plastica 111
lithotripsy 222
liver 128
lobar pneumonia 9, 16
looser zones 246
lymphangiography 146
lymphatic system anatomy 144

mal union of fractures 275-6
malabsorption syndrome 120
mammary dysplasia 148
Mantoux test 22-3
marble bone disease: *see* osteopetrosis
March fracture 294
measles 10, 26
meconium ileus 28
mediastinal masses 41-2
medullary sponge kidney 207-8
medulloblastoma 186
megacolon 113, 119, 123
melanoma 192, 197-8
membranous lupus nephritis 210
Menière's disease 189
meningioma 186
meningitis 21, 173-6
meningocoele 163
meningomyelocoele 163
mesothelioma 33
microcephaly 158
micturition 229, 282
miliary tuberculosis, 21, 176
mitral valve disease 62-4
Monteggia fracture 287
motor neurone disease 182
mouth anatomy 97
mucoviscidosis: *see* cystic fibrosis
multiple sclerosis 178-80
mumps 10, 176
muscle anatomy 200-201
muscular atrophy 202
muscular dystrophy 201-202
myasthenia gravis 201
myeloma 183, 254-5, 277
myelosclerosis 247
myocardial infarction (MI) 60-61
myxoedema 68, 305

nasopharynx anatomy 11
nebuliser 30
neurofibroma 183, 186-7, 255
neurofibromatosis 187
neuropathic joints: *see* Charcot joints
non-Hodgkin's lymphoma 147
non-union of fractures 272
nose anatomy 11

oat cell carcinoma 40, 41
obstruction 106, 117, 123, 124, 126, 230
occupational lung disease 32-33
oesophagitis 103-4
oesophagus anatomy 102
    atresia and stenosis 102
oligodendroglioma 185
Ollier's disease 250
oral monoliasis 99
orchidectomy 234
Osgood-Schlatter disease 259
osteoblastoma 253, 254
osteochondritis dissecan 259
osteogenesis imperfecta 244, 277
osteoma 252
osteomalacia 245-6
osteomyelitis 9, 248-50, 273
osteopenia 243
osteopetrosis 247
osteoporosis 31, 243-44, 277, 311
osteosarcoma 248, 252-3
osteosclerosis 247-8
otitis media 177, 189
ovary anatomy 239

Paget's disease 183, 247-8
Pancoast's tumour 40, 41
pancreas anatomy 138
pancreatitis 139, 142
papillary necrosis 213-14, 221
papilloedema 191
papilloma 149
paralytic ileus 123
paranasal sinuses anatomy 11-12
    sinusitis 12
paraplegia 183, 229-30, 281-2
parathyroid anatomy 306-7
Parkinson's disease 177, 180-81
patent ductus arteriosus (PDA) 53-4
pathological fractures 276-7
pathology 1
pelvic osteotomy 257
peptic ulcer 108-10
perforation 126
peripheral nervous system 156
peritoneum 127, 143
peritonitis 126, 127

Perthes' disease 258-9
petit mal 188
phaeochromocytoma 69, 227, 313
pinealoma 187
pituitary gland anatomy 295-7
pituitary tumour 300
platelets 95
platybasia 164
pleiomorphic adenoma 101-2
pleura 42-3
pleural effusion 15, 21, 41, 43
pleural thickening 43
pleurodesis 37
pneumoconioses 32
pneumonia 15-17, 21, 30, 275
pneumothorax 15, 26, 30, 33-7
poliomyelitis 176
polyarthritis 61, 62
polyarteritis nodosa 183
polycystic disease 69
polycystic kidney 208-9
polycythaemia 81-2
polyps 125
    endometrial 237, 238
    large intestine 125
    paranasal sinuses 12
    stomach 112
polyuria 139, 299, 308
positron emission tomography (PET) 181
post-primary tuberculosis 21
post traumatic ossification 276
Pott's fracture 263, 292-3
pre-eclampsia 70
pressure sores 274
primary tuberculosis 21
progressive bulbar palsy 182
progressive massive fibrosis (PMF): see
    pneumoconioses
progressive muscular atrophy 182
prolapsed bladder 230
prolapsed vertebral disc 182
prostate gland enlargement 232-3
proteinurea 205
pseudopolyps 125
pulmonary embolism 37-8, 274
pulmonary emphysema 25-6
pulmonary stenosis 54
pulmonary valvotomy 55
purified protein derivative (PPD) 22

pyelonephritis 213
pyloric stenosis 108
pyopneumothorax 37

radiological union 271
Rashkind procedure 57
Reiter's disease 262
renal dialysis 211, 216-18, 255
renal failure 215-16, 224
renal length 204
renal transplant 218-20
retinoblastoma 191
retinopathy 141
rheumatic fever 61-2, 66
rheumatic heart disease 61
rhinitis 11, 12
rhinovirus 11
rickets 245
rodent ulcer 196
rubella 10, 50, 190
rudimentary heart 49-50

salbutamol 30
salivary glands 100-102
sarcoidosis 31-2, 248
sciatica 183
Scribner shunt 217
scurvy 244
secondary tumours 3, 5, 6, 40, 41, 73,
    126, 137, 147, 150, 186-7, 197-8, 226,
    233, 236, 238, 254, 255, 306
seminoma 235
septicaemia 9
sequestrum 273
Sever's disease 259
Sheehan's syndrome 298
shingles 177
shunts 160-1
sialodenitis 100
sialolithiasis 100
sickle cell anaemia 87-9, 248
sinusitis 12
skin anatomy 194
skip lesions 114
slipped femoral epiphysis 259-60
Smith's fracture 288
spina bifida 162

spinal cord anatomy 153
spondylisthesis 165, 279
sputum 15, 27, 53
St Vitus' dance: *see* Sydenham's chorea
stagnant bowel syndrome 124
status asthmaticus 30
steatorrhoea 29, 120
Steinmann pin 273
Still's disease 262
stomach anatomy 107
subacute bacterial endocarditis (SBE) 9
subarachnoid haemmorhage (SAH) 67,
   166-7, 173
supracondylar fracture 286
surgical emphysema 24-5
Sydenham's chorea 61
synovial joint anatomy 256-7
syphilis 50
syringomyelocoele 164
systemic lupus erythematosis (SLE) 199-
   200, 210

tachycardia 71
teratoma 42, 236
testes anatomy 235
tetanus 274
thalassaemia 89-90
thrombocytaemia 82
thrombocytopenia 95-6
thrombophlebitis 75
thyroid gland anatomy 301-302
thyrotoxicosis 68
tine test 22-3
tophi 263
Tokildsen's operation 161
trans-ischaemic attack (TIA) 168-9
transposition of great vessels 57
transudate 42
transverse cardiac diameter 46
tricuspid valve disease 66
trimalleolar fracture 293
tuberculin test 21
tuberculosis 9, 183, 214-15,
   bone 250
   joint 263
tumour:
   acinar carcinoma 143
   acoustic neuroma 189-90

adrenal gland 227
bile duct 133
bone 251-4
bone marrow 254-5
breast 149-52
bronchus 39-41
carcinoid tumour 124
cartilage 253
cervix 238
characteristics 2-3
classification 3-5
definition 2
endometrium 238
floor of mouth 100
gall bladder 133
grading 6
heart 73
hepatoblastoma 137
Hodgkin's 145-7
Islet cell tumour 142
intestine 125-7
kidney 225-7
liver 137
Krukenberg's 112
larynx 13
lip 98
mediastinum 41-2
melanoma 197-8
methods of spread 5-6
nervous system 184-7
non-Hodgkin's lymphoma 147
oesophagus 107
ovary 239-40
Pancoast's 40, 41
pancreas 142-3
pericardium 73
peritoneum 127
pituitary 300-301
prostate 233
rodent ulcer 196
salivary gland 101
seminoma 235-6
stomach 111
teratoma 42, 236
thyroid 42, 306
tongue 99
skin 195-6
Turner's syndrome 240
typhoid fever 9

Index

ulcerative colitis 117-19, 123
uraemia 205
urethra anatomy 234, 240
urethral stricture 234
urethritis 234
urinary bladder 227
urinary tract infection (UTI) 208, 212-15, 221
urodynamics 229
urticaria 81, 135
uterine fibroids: *see* leiomyomas
uterus anatomy 236

vagotomy 110
varices 75, 106
varicose veins 75
venesection 81
ventolin 30
ventricular septal defect (VSD) 52-3, 70
ventricular tachycardia (VT) 72

verruca 195
Virchow's node 112
virus:
    Epstein-barr 147
    general 10
    German measles 50
    herpes zoster 176, 177
    mumps 176
    pneumonia 15
    viral hepatitis 133
    volvulus 122, 123
von Recklinghausen's disease 246
von Willebrand's disease 91-2

Wallerian degeneration 183
Waterston operation 57
whiplash injury 278
whooping cough 26
Wilm's tumour 226
Wolff-Parkinson-White syndrome 72